"Dr. Sarah LoBisco, ND, has provided a useful and timely look at today's healthcare by referencing both allopathic and holistic approaches in her book BreakFree Medicine: A Systematic and Integrative Guide to Balancing the Body. Many are choosing to move away from the allopathic approaches of prescription drugs, surgeries, and aggressive medical treatments as remedies for their medical concerns. The challenge becomes one of where to find accurate information concerning more holistic and integrative treatments. Dr. LoBisco has solved that problem by providing a practical and accurate guide that will benefit the modern day healthcare consumer.

I am thrilled to be a follower of Dr. LoBisco's blog and newsletter. She is passionate about researching and sharing the most up-to-date professional information on all things holistic. Her book is a welcome extension to her work. It will guide us to better understand the variety of modern healthcare options and benefits available to restore our vibrant health."

-Carol Lovelee, MA, Certified Integrative Energy Practitioner, author of Tears to Giggles

"Dr. LoBisco has collected information from a vast array of experts in the field of alternative medicine and distilled it into a way of living that is not only science-based, but is practical, easy to implement, cost-effective and imminently logical. In short, we have more than enough books on alternative medicine. What are desperately lacking are books that make it easy for everyone to incorporate alternative medicine into their everyday lives. For those people who want to go beyond interest and actually use alternative medicine to create a happy and healthy life, this book is a must read."

-Jeffrey Moss, DDS, CNS, DACBN, Moss Nutrition Products, Inc.

BreakFree Medicine

A Systematic and Integrative
Guide to Balancing Your Body

Sarah LoBisco, ND

BALBOA
PRESS
A DIVISION OF HAY HOUSE

Copyright © 2016 Sarah A LoBisco, ND.

Headshot photo © 2016 Blackburn Portrait Design

All rights reserved. No part of this book may be used or reproduced by any means, graphic, electronic, or mechanical, including photocopying, recording, taping or by any information storage retrieval system without the written permission of the author except in the case of brief quotations embodied in critical articles and reviews.

Balboa Press books may be ordered through booksellers or by contacting:

Balboa Press
A Division of Hay House
1663 Liberty Drive
Bloomington, IN 47403
www.balboapress.com
1 (877) 407-4847

Because of the dynamic nature of the Internet, any web addresses or links contained in this book may have changed since publication and may no longer be valid. The views expressed in this work are solely those of the author and do not necessarily reflect the views of the publisher, and the publisher hereby disclaims any responsibility for them.

This book is intended for information and educational purposes only. It is not intended to diagnose, treat, or prescribe for any condition or replace direct clinical management with a qualified healthcare practitioner. The author or the publisher shall not be liable or responsible for any consequence of your use or application of any information or suggestions in this book.

Any people depicted in stock imagery provided by Thinkstock are models, and such images are being used for illustrative purposes only. Certain stock imagery © Thinkstock.

Print information available on the last page.

ISBN: 978-1-4525-1748-3 (sc)
ISBN: 978-1-4525-1750-6 (hc)
ISBN: 978-1-4525-1749-0 (e)

Library of Congress Control Number: 2014911441

Balboa Press rev. date: 02/19/2016

DEDICATION

To my family- Mom, Dad, Kate, Jeff, Anna, Hank, and Mo. Thank you all for shining so brightly; it is through your light and support that I have the courage to shine mine.

EPIGRAPH

"If I have seen a little further it is by standing on the shoulders of Giants."

-Newton's remark to Hooke in 1676

CONTENTS

Foreword xiii
Preface.. xv
Acknowledgements xix
Introduction xxi
    A New Viewpoint on Healthcare xxii
        The Art of Medicine xxii
        The Business of Medicine xxii

Chapter 1 - Traditional, Conventional, and Natural Medicine:
                The Power of a Beautiful Integration 1
    Today's Conventional Medicine Statistics 2
    Room for Improvement 6
    The Problem with Known "Truths" in Medicine 7
        For the Love of Pseudoscience and Medicine 9
        Using a Model of Control in an Uncontrollable World 11
    But ... Is Natural Medicine Really Safe? 14

Chapter 2 - A New Approach to Individualized Treatment 16
    Shifting the Outlook on "Wellness" 17
        Searching for a Miracle Pill 19
        A More Individualized Approach to Medicine 20
    Biochemistry: Honoring Your Unique Makeup 24
    All Systems Go ... Together 26
    Looking Forward 27

Chapter 3 - Let Food Be Thy Medicine 30
    Start with a Positive Outlook 31
    Biochemical Imbalances Result in Cravings 33
    Easing Into Healthy Food Choices: Balancing the Body 34
        Tuning In 35
        Your Perfect Diet: Embrace Your Individuality! 36
    Pass Up the Gluten 38
        What About Wheat in Another Form? 41
        The Benefits of a Gluten-Free Mood 42
        How to Go Gluten-Free 44
    The Sweetness of Life? Reconsidering Sugar 45
    The Case for and Against Soy 46
    And Then We Have the Super-Supplements… 49
    What to Eat? Let's Make This Simple 50

Chapter 4 - Moving Toward Healthier Outcomes.............................52
    Weight Loss the Integrative Way 54
    What About Genes (not Jeans)? 56
    Lead Your Own Weigh! 57
    The Best (Blood) Type of Workout? 59
    Debunking the All-Inclusive Use of the Latest Trend 62
    Don't Forget … Love Yourself 64

Chapter 5 - Your Gut: The Home of Mood, Food, and Immunity.......67
    Leaky Gut 69
    Different People, Different Causes 72
    System-Wide Breakdowns 72
        Celiac Disease versus Gluten Sensitivity 77
        Moderation is Key 80
    Probiotics 80
        The Bottom Line on Probiotic Supplements 82
    Tips for a Healthy Gastrointestinal Tract 83

Chapter 6 - Healthy Body, Healthy Brain.. 85
    The Conventional Approach to Depression 86
    A Pill for the Mentally Ill 88
    Why Drugs Are Missing the Mark 92
    A More Integrated Approach to Treating Depression 94
    Looking into the Brain 96
        The Link for All Brain Functions 107
    Remember, You're Not in This Alone 112

Chapter 7 - Finding Hormonal Harmony... 113
    Hormones Off Balance 114
    The Importance of Testing & the Caveats 115
    The Thyroid Connection... 118
    Stressed-Out Hormones 119
        More On the "Numbing" Effects of Stress 121
        Sex Hormone Shifts... 123
        Menopause... 125
        Key Factors for Hormonal Health.. 125
    Hormone Replacement Therapy 128
    Find a Happy Balance 130

Chapter 8 - Toxic in the 21st Century 131
    So Why Isn't Everyone Sick? 132
    Toxic Bodies and Toxic Fat.. 134
        What to Consider When Cleansing.. 136
        The Importance of Clean Eating in a Dirty World 138
        Tips for Making Our Bodies Safe in a Scary World................. 140
        Dirty Energy 143
    Emotional Toxicity 145
    Putting It All Together: Holistic and Comprehensive
        Support for Cleansing and Toxicity... 147
        Healthy Detoxing in a Partnership of Support....................... 147

Chapter 9 - Heart & Soul Medicine 149
    The Flaws in Treating Every Heart Ill with a Pill 152
    Beyond Numbers for Heart Health 153
        Emotional Heart Health 154

Chapter 10 - Conclusion 156
    Moving Forward with This Book 156

Epilogue 159
About the Author 161
Glossary 163
Resources: for Further Reading 167
References by Chapter 169
Index 193

FOREWORD

Dr. Sarah LoBisco, a gifted naturopathic physician and respected colleague, has done a masterful job at explaining the extremely complex subject of how our healthcare system is failing us and what logical steps can be taken to avert a national public health and financial disaster. She confronts head-on the controversies that swirl around the modern medical profession, including the undue influences of the pharmaceutical and insurance industries, the almost exclusive use of toxic substances, otherwise known as drugs, as a first-line intervention when other, less risky options are widely available and proven. She also summarizes the political and economic issues at play in preventing consumers from knowing the entire truth about the risks involved when going to see a conventional physician. Dr. LoBisco also eloquently makes the case for "whole-body" health, as practiced by the modern licensed naturopathic and functional medicine physician, and her commitment as a doctor to treat her clients as whole human beings and not just a gastrointestinal tract, a heart, or other organ or system, is clearly apparent. Within this context, she tackles many difficult issues, including the role of stress, lifestyle, diet, toxins, emotions and attitudes in health and disease. If you are suffering from chronic poor health, this book is a must-read. It will allow you to understand all the complex factors that may be playing a role in your condition, and it will prepare you to serve as a knowledgeable self-advocate with your physicians and healthcare providers, who often do not recognize, nor appreciate, all of these associated factors. It will help you understand all of your options, and not just the ones generally presented to you by standard physicians who do not practice from an enlightened perspective.

Sincerely,

David M. Brady, ND, CCN, DACBN
Vice Provost, Health Sciences Division
Director, Human Nutrition Institute
Associate Professor of Clinical Sciences
University of Bridgeport (Bridgeport, CT)
Private Practice: Whole Body Medicine (Trumbull, CT)

PREFACE

As I began my journey in healthcare, I was saddened to learn that there seemed to be two opposing viewpoints of medicine in our society. "Real" medicine consisted of a standard of care, conventional approach that was taught in the educational institutions of medical doctors and primary care providers. The main modality taught was the use of pharmaceuticals. Any other approach outside this standard was considered second-best and labeled as "pseudoscience" at worst, or viewed as an "alternative" or "complementary" therapy at best.

In my three years of working as a pharmacy technician, I witnessed firsthand the power and limitations of relying on only one method of treatment for every individual. Though helpful when properly prescribed, the sole utilization of powerful drugs as the main component of disease management hasn't proven to be a cure for the chronic diseases that plague our globe today. Even our most powerful "magic bullet" antibiotics are becoming obsolete, based on the alarming rise in microorganisms now resistant to them. Thankfully, the tides in healing seem to be changing.

More and more, complementary and alternative therapies, which are truly traditional in practice, are being validated as effective and safe modalities for wellness. I have written this book as a guide for those who are seeking scientifically sound, safe, and integrative solutions to common and chronic health conditions. *BreakFree Medicine* is for both patients and practitioners alike who desire holistic wellness solutions beyond symptom control or the use of another pill that may create more side effects. It provides techniques and tools that assist everyone to live the healthiest possible life through a combination of naturopathic and functional healing modalities.

Although the tools for healing can differ between conventional and integrative medicine, the intention to heal the sufferer remains the same. It is my hope that this book will help you cast aside the fear and false belief that disease is something to wage war against. Instead, I invite you to discover your own innate healing capacity and to regard distressing symptoms as information from your body that, when decoded, helps point to solutions that fully restore your health.

Sarah LoBisco, ND Doctor of Naturopathic Medicine

Naturopathic Physician's Oath

I dedicate myself to the service of humanity as a practitioner of the art and science of Naturopathic medicine. I will honor my teachers and all who have preserved and developed this knowledge, and dedicate myself to supporting the growth and evolution of Naturopathic medicine.

I will endeavor to continually improve my abilities as a healer through study, reflection, and genuine concern for humanity.

I will impart knowledge of the advanced healing arts to dedicated colleagues and students.

Through precept, lecture, and example, I will assist and encourage others to strengthen their health, reduce risks of disease, and preserve the health of our planet for our families, our future generations, and ourselves.

According to my best ability and judgment, I will use methods of treatment, which follow the principles of Naturopathic medicine:

- First of all, to do no harm.
- To act in cooperation with the healing power of nature.
- To address the fundamental causes of disease.
- To heal the whole person through individualized treatment.
- To teach the principles of healthy living and preventive medicine.

I will conduct my life and the practice of Naturopathic healthcare with vigilance, integrity, and freedom from prejudice.

I will abstain from voluntary acts of injustice and corruption. I will keep confidential whatever I am privileged to witness, whether professionally or privately, that should not be divulged.

With my whole heart, before this gathering of witnesses, as a doctor of Naturopathic medicine, I pledge to remain true to this oath.

ACKNOWLEDGEMENTS

I'd like to thank ...

My family: Without them, I couldn't do what I do.

My friends and guides for supporting me: Matt Laughlin, Faith, Caron, Marion, Sherry, and Reisa.

My esteemed colleagues and medical mentors: Dr. David Brady, Dr. Jeffrey Moss, and Dr. Richard Herbold.

God/Universe/Spirit: for guidance and playing his/her song through me in medicine and writing.

Robert Holden and the Hay House authors: for their wisdom and guidance.

Terry Quigley: for her patience in helping me with proofreading, her belief in my ability to be the change I wish to bring to healthcare, and for being my mom and one of my best friends.

Dr. Mary James: for her superb medical editing and attention to detail.

Shelly Hagen: for her assistance in compiling, organizing, and assisting with my original content.

Danielle Klahr: for her initial editing support.

Balboa Press and Adriane Pontecorvo: for their kindness, patience, and dedication to making this book project transform into an authentic reality.

INTRODUCTION

A VOICE FOR CHANGE IN MEDICINE

We live in a world where aggression and domination seem to be prominent in every aspect of society, even in medicine. We declare war, not just on people, but also on diseases, theologies, and viewpoints. There is a "war on cancer," a "war on AIDS," and even a "war on healthcare reform." There is a bombardment of fear in the media, which cites disease outbreaks and the aggressive measures taken to "fight" and "eradicate" them. Instead of celebrating our bodies and honoring our intuition, we succumb to fear and rely on extreme measures to suppress their signals. This fear-based system has created a multi-million dollar industry, not to mention exhausted physicians and unsatisfied patients.

In this new merger between business and medicine, resulting in the additional burden of responsibility of insurance processing, patient quotas, demands for quick results for "consumers," and electronic health records, even the most dedicated physician can become jaded. Practitioners must find their own comfort level while seeking balance between practicing their art and the business of the bottom line. I have been witness to some unfortunate misaligned results ... bleeding hearts are forced out of practice or unsatisfied patients are treated as price tags. I believe in a better way.

A New Viewpoint on Healthcare

The Art of Medicine

My journey in healing has led me to a viewpoint in medicine that embraces integration between the innate intelligence of the body, a reverence for its divine manifestation, and a loyalty to optimize and support its biology. I have found that there is no war that must be won between health and disease. "Fighting" disease does not work with the body. If we balance the body by supplying it with all that it needs (physical, emotional, and spiritual), replace what it is lacking, and remove physical or emotional stressors, restoration will result. At that point, we can focus on how to stay well.

The Business of Medicine

When the body is optimized, so too are the mind and the spirit. This is my definition of holism. As consumers get more in tune with their own innate wellness as an inborn and authentic quality, they will be more willing to prioritize their health. Investing in their own wellness and consulting specialists who work with this philosophy (e.g., functional medicine practitioners, naturopathic doctors) will rate as highly as purchasing a cruise or the latest technological device, for example.

The demand for high-quality healthcare, along with an insistence on the re-unification of the body, mind, and soul, will create a shift in how medicine is practiced. This form of holism will occur, not as a national riot, in which sides form and battle for better insurance coverage, but through one patient-doctor relationship at a time.

Eventually, a new system of healthcare will emerge that is tailored to each individual. This can only be accomplished through reclaiming our own power to choose and refusing to allow a third party to decide how to "reimburse" our healthcare decisions.

My vision and prayer is to become part of a healthcare environment in which patients thrive, not just survive.

CHAPTER 1

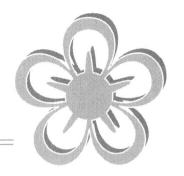

Traditional, Conventional, and Natural Medicine: The Power of a Beautiful Integration

Naturopathic doctors revere the body's innate ability to heal and to be restored to optimal function through the least invasive, most natural means possible. This philosophy views disease as a state of imbalance, and believes that when the body is provided with what it needs, it is restored to its natural balance. Our aim is to address the underlying cause of disease, remove any obstacles to cure, and support the body with the proper nourishment it needs to heal.

My training in naturopathic philosophy has been furthered by the study of functional medicine, which provides insight into one's unique biochemistry. It utilizes a holistic model that incorporates specific biological assessments to help determine individualized nutritional needs and deficiencies. Functional medicine also offers insight into how various supplements or medications affect each person's body differently.

Conventional medicine, which is the medicine practiced by today's medical doctors (MDs) and their allied professionals, tends to rely more on tools aimed at covering or suppressing symptoms. Although I am trained in the use of pharmaceuticals and diagnostic tools of modern and scientific research, I have earned the letters "ND" (vs. "MD") after my name because of the ways in which I use, apply, and view those tools. This book is not meant to assert which type of medicine is better. Both are needed. I have the utmost respect for conventional medical practitioners and their brilliance. I am not questioning their abilities, diagnostic excellence, or knowledge of core clinical sciences. I do, however, agree with most of my colleagues who use integrative medicine. Conventional medicine tends to apply this knowledge by suppressing symptoms without always addressing causes... an approach that could be contributing to today's healthcare crisis.

Today's Conventional Medicine Statistics

Many people who are interested in healthcare reform and integrative medicine are familiar with Gary Null's publication, *Death by Medicine*, a compilation of various studies on the state of healthcare statistics in the United States.[1] This publication cites sources for estimated costs, death rates, and unnecessary medical events. Null lists the following conditions with an estimated rate of mortality that totals 7,841,360:

>	Adverse drug reactions
>	Medical errors
>	Bedsores
>	Nosocomial (hospital-based) infections
>	Malnutrition
>	Outpatient errors
>	Unnecessary procedures
>	Surgery-related complications

Null concludes, "Our estimated 10-year total of 7.8 million iatrogenic [a condition unintentionally caused by the actions or words of a physician] deaths is more than all the casualties from all the wars fought by the US throughout its entire history."[1] Yikes! This is quite an alarming conclusion for most of us to hear, especially since we are led to believe that we have one of the best healthcare systems in the world.

Recently, I came across an updated statistic on our country's dreary healthcare outcomes. A meta-analysis[2] in the September 2013 issue of the *Journal of Patient Safety* affirmed "that a lower limit of 210,000 deaths per year was associated with preventable harm in hospitals," with an upper limit of approximately 400,000. Interestingly, this analysis was limited to only four studies and only took into consideration specific medical harms using the Global Trigger Tool to flag specific evidence in medical records.

A June 2010 report[3] by the Commonwealth Fund, a private organization advocating for a "high performance health care system providing better access, improved quality, and greater efficiency," echoed Null's disconcerting news on the state of US healthcare. As stated in the Executive Summary of their 34-page report,

> *The U.S. health system is the most expensive in the world, but comparative analyses consistently show the United States underperforms relative to other countries on most dimensions of performance. This report, which includes information from the most recent three Commonwealth Fund surveys of patients and primary care physicians about medical practices and views of their countries' health systems (2007-2009), confirms findings discussed in previous editions of Mirror, Mirror. It also includes information on health care outcomes that were featured in the most recent (2008) U.S. health system scorecard issued by the Commonwealth Fund Commission on a High Performance Health System.*[3]

Among the seven nations of Australia, Canada, Germany, the Netherlands, New Zealand, the United States, and the United Kingdom (UK), the United States ranked last in overall health outcomes. The United States has also ranked last in the 2004, 2006, and 2007 editions. The Netherlands, UK, and Australia scored highest in patient and physician survey results for the experience and dimensions of care. The following items were among the considerations for key findings in this report:

1. Quality of care and access
2. Efficiency
3. Equity
4. Quality of life

It is concerning that the United States fails to achieve better results for healthcare, falling behind seven nations in the dimensions of access, patient safety, coordination, efficiency, and equity. Universal health coverage was absent in the United States, which was a notable difference from the other countries. Furthermore, the other six countries spent less money per person and overall in healthcare's gross national product compared to the United States. It is questionable whether President Barack Obama's healthcare reform legislation will improve affordability and access in the future. During the editing of this book, The Common Wealth Fund released their 2015 report, "U.S. Health Care from a Global Perspective: Spending, Use of Services, Prices, and Health in 13 Countries" and reported similar results in 2013 as in 2010, stating that, "Despite spending more on health care, Americans had poor health outcomes, including shorter life expectancy and greater prevalence of chronic conditions."

Ten years after The Institute of Medicine issued their article, "To Err is Human," a 2010 study examined possible harms to hospital admissions in North Carolina between 2002 and 2007. The report,[4] published in the *New England Journal of Medicine*, suggested that the above statistics concerning medication errors and conventional treatments are not improving:

> In a study of 10 North Carolina hospitals, we found that harms remain common, with little evidence of widespread improvement. Further efforts are needed to translate effective safety interventions into routine practice and to monitor health care safety over time.[4]

A 2006 analysis from the *Journal of the American Medical Association* found that 21,298 adverse drug events in emergency rooms were reported by an estimated 701,547 individuals in a two-year span.[5] Among these cases, 3,487 required hospitalization. Drugs requiring regular outpatient monitoring in order to prevent acute toxicity were responsible for 41.5 percent of the estimated hospitalizations overall.

According to a 2010 review, adverse drug reactions (ADRs) are of special concern for those over 65, females, and young children.[6] The authors stated that in emergency departments, ADRs were found more frequently in elderly patients who were on multiple medications and who had more than one diagnosis. In children, it was estimated that 5.4 percent had ADRs, with 56.7 percent of these being related to beta-lactam antibiotics. Of concern, only 6.9 percent of children with ADRs were referred for further investigation.

This review also noted that among children suffering from an immune-related blood disorder, there were associations between selected antibiotics, anti-inflammatory medications, mucolytics, and measles, mumps, and rubella (MMR) vaccination. Finally, female gender was a factor in developing ADRs, in general, and atopy (a type of allergic hypersensitivity response), was a risk factor for beta-lactam antibiotic sensitization in female hospital nurses.

Room for Improvement

Depressing news, isn't it? Or is it? Despite some of the negative press around doctors and healthcare, I never cease to be amazed at the absolute dedication and brilliance of professionals across all medical specialties. I believe that most doctors wish to do what is best for the patient, based on what they are taught. Physicians come into this profession to help people, not to hurt them. The fact that we are not doing well with outcomes simply indicates that there is room for change.

The answer lies in a new approach, one that uses a blend of conventional, integrative, functional, and naturopathic medicine. Instead of depending on the acute care model to treat chronic diseases, this approach shifts the focus to lifestyle and diet modifications to prevent them. It unites the science of epigenetics, nutrigenomics, individualized supplementation, and mind-body techniques.

This new viewpoint reflects a very different mindset than the "pill for every ill" mentality of conventional medicine. Although appropriate for traumatic or acute conditions, our current quick-fix mindset for long-term health has led us to the pathetic statistics I listed earlier in this chapter. It teaches people to ignore and suppress their bodies' warning signs with magic pills until we are barreling right through stop signs toward a major crash-and-burn. The result is a disconnect between the body, mind, and spirit, and a potential strain in the patient-doctor relationship.

Thankfully, there is a new approach which solves this problem using a completely different model. I will dive more into this model in Chapter 2. The good news is that we don't need to change all the tools at our disposal, just how and when we use them. This approach applies integrative methods to empower the patient and to help achieve the highest level of health for every individual.

The Problem with Known "Truths" in Medicine

You may be wondering why a book on natural medicine is turning into a discussion of philosophy, but the two are quite interconnected. A strong tie between healing and psychology has been noted since the beginning of time. The father of medicine, Hippocrates, said, "It is more important to know what sort of person has a disease than to know what sort of disease a person has." Many can relate only too well to this statement. I hear my clients exclaim time and time again that they wish their conventional doctors would simply listen to them. It is a simple request, yet why is it so hard to come by?

In the current economy, doctors who wish to assess psychological contributors to their clients' symptoms are also faced with the practical business ramifications of running a practice in which payment is typically not reimbursed for such "frivolities." According to the American Medical Association (AMA), physician reimbursement is based on three factors:

> *In 1992, the federal government established a standardized Medicare physician payment schedule based on a resource-based relative value scale (RBRVS). Under this scale, physician service payments are calculated based upon the cost of the service provided as divided into three components: physician work, practice expense and professional liability insurance.*[7]

This approach brings attention to the fact that we are not suffering from a lack of knowledgeable and brilliant medical minds; rather, the payment model does not allow for integrity, authenticity, and courage.

There is a sense in medicine that "healing" is based more on insurance premiums and the bottom line of the pharmaceutical industry than on physicians making treatment decisions based on the individual patient.

It seems that the ultimate authority regarding coverage of services are the insurance companies. Dr. Kirsch expresses his frustration in being caught in this model where clear ethical boundaries are indistinct:

> When I select a specialist for a patient, I first look at the patient's list of approved physicians instead of immediately suggesting the best available specialist. If a patient needs to be hospitalized, then I must know which hospitals are in the insurance company's network. And when a pharmacy calls me because my choice of a medicine is not on the patient's formulary, I casually prescribe another medication.[8]

Kirsch is brave enough to acknowledge the possibility of hypocrisy of physicians practicing at their highest ability within a system run by the business of insurance companies. This seems to be true even among doctors who claim to practice high ethical standards. For example, it is not uncommon for physicians to be guided in their choices of labs and imaging based on a patient's insurance plan. Furthermore, insurance companies are in the position of determining which medications are covered and whether a patient can afford a physician's first choice of what to prescribe.

Although the new approach to medicine described in this book promises better outcomes, the *business* of medicine makes the acceptance of it slow in coming. Preventative medicine and long-term goals are up against human nature's desire for the quick fix and that alluring quest to discover THE cure, THE diet, THE pill, or THE miracle. In today's society, advertisers and marketers have convinced us that their particular panacea will produce fast and effortless results, and with money-back guarantees. We are bombarded by the media's brilliant catering to this primitive, gluttonous quest. The use of mindless brainwashing techniques, empty promises, and a "pill for every ill" as the instantaneous answer are the solutions offered, regardless of how many years of abuse our body has been through.

These messages produce a cultural norm to pop a pill, erase the symptoms, and keep on going. This presents a challenge for those in the integrative health fields. Naturopathic doctors, whose philosophy incorporates finding the true *cause* of a disease or symptom, not instant fixes, can be easily drowned out by the millions of dollars spent on advertising quick cure-alls with sexy marketing campaigns. It is, indeed, a sad state of affairs when money is not just the bottom line of Ebenezer Scrooge cronies, but also the final say in how we heal. What is most disappointing and scary to me is that when I receive inquiries for my service, the first question is typically, "Does insurance cover your services?" It reflects the modern viewpoint that healthcare comes down to the best deal. How sad! And how infuriating to both doctors and patients! Society has trained the sick to regard their healing as a commodity to the best bidder. Oh, Judas!

In this book, I am inviting you to slow down and awaken to that quiet, calm voice within. This voice will lead you into a healing partnership with your doctor, not encourage a split between you and your body. In the next section, I will invite you to question your belief about science and explain to you why our current model is lacking.

For the Love of Pseudoscience and Medicine

I love medicine and I love science. That's why I studied to become a naturopathic doctor. I know there is room for both. Here's the thing, though ... science isn't the ultimate truth. Rather, science is a system of knowledge that covers certain truths. Merriam-Webster defines science as...

1. : the state of knowing: knowledge as distinguished from ignorance or misunderstanding
2. a: a department of systematized knowledge as an object of study <the science of theology>
   b: something (as a sport or technique) that may be studied or learned like systematized knowledge <have it down to a science>
3. a: knowledge or a system of knowledge covering general truths or the operation of general laws especially as obtained and tested through scientific method
   b: such knowledge or such a system of knowledge concerned with the physical world and its phenomena: natural science
4. : a system or method reconciling practical ends with scientific laws <cooking is both a science and an art>

When we look at the definition of science with an open mind, the question of whether science is indeed a theology in itself is a valid one. Some might view this as blasphemy, but today's science is mostly based within the confines of testing the theories of other scientists and proving or disproving their methods. In this instance, we are claiming that what is to be considered true is only in what has been previously explored. That's why the whole definition of science can be misleading when "breakthroughs" occur or a different viewpoint on conventional science is expressed. The truth is, if it cannot be explained within the confines of current understanding, the majority of society views it as a threat. Unfortunately, this means that the very subject of natural health can be threatening to our current view of medicine because it isn't what is currently accepted within the definition of the "science of medicine." According to an article in *The Humanist*, science may indeed be a form of religion:

> In its pure form, science is supposed to be used for exploration and discovery, not for conforming and confirming what is already present. The fact is Science

> is becoming a political, economic, and theological basis in which anything beyond status quo and conventional thinking is looked upon as pseudo-science or dangerous. It makes me question, has science become a fundamentalist religion?[9]

Using a Model of Control in an Uncontrollable World

When assessing the impact of natural healing modalities, the use of this linear, evidence-based model (EBM) of reasoning falls short. The concept of the EBM is based on the idea that in a specific, controlled environment, one, and only one, intervention is responsible for producing a positive or negative effect compared to a given placebo treatment. The results are compiled and peer-reviewed, and confounding factors (such as experimenter bias and expectations of participants) are controlled for. Based on the strength of the design model, sample size, and clinical efficacy, clinicians use these results to tweak their therapeutic protocols.

In an audio presentation[10] from the *Natural Medicine Journal*, I listened to various clinical experts address the subject of the use of evidence-based medicine for assessing efficacy of treatments used in nutritional and plant-based medicine. The speakers were asked to discuss the pros and pitfalls of using a conventional model of assessment in natural medicine. Disregarding the lack of appropriate funding, there is a variety of issues that arise when using this model to assess the efficacy of medical interventions, in general, and even more so for natural medicine.[10]

> Issue 1: Most clinicians don't find these outcome studies to be relevant to their *clinical* practice, or they don't have the time and training required to properly review the articles and interpret the results independent of the researcher's conclusions. Because of this, they rely on summaries from drug companies

or other biased sources that may prioritize sales over healing and what's best for the patient. This leads to issue number 2...

Issue 2: Data is usually skewed in favor of the company funding the study. The *British Medical Journal* article "Clinical Evidence"[11] analyzed common medical treatments that are supported by sufficient reliable evidence. The investigators reviewed approximately 2,500 treatments and found that only 13 percent were considered beneficial. Among the remainder, 23 percent were "likely to be beneficial," 8 percent were likely to be equally harmful or beneficial, 6 percent were not likely to be helpful, and 4 percent were likely to be harmful or ineffective. Interestingly, almost half, or 46 percent, were unknown to be useful or injurious.

Issue 3: In real life, people are not in a controlled environment where confounding factors are removed and only one medication is used. According to classical homeopath, Dana Ullman, who commented on the above study,

> Today in America, every man, woman, and child is prescribed around 13 prescription drugs per year (and this doesn't count the many over-the-counter drugs that doctors prescribe and that patients take on their own). Just 12 years earlier, Americans were on average prescribed less than eight drugs per person, a 62 percent increase! The fact of the matter is that drugs are not tested for approval in conjunction with other drugs, and the safety and efficacy of the use of multiple drugs together remains totally unknown ... According to a 2008 nationwide survey, 29 percent of Americans used at least five prescription medications concurrently.[12]

Issue 4: The concept of *hormesis* is usually omitted in clinical trials. A constituent found in a plant can have therapeutic, neutral, or toxic effects depending on how it's used in the body and the level of imbalance in the body. This concept makes it hard to translate evidence-based models, used in randomized, placebo-controlled studies, to an interactive model that takes into account synergistic effects and the state of the individual.

Issue 5: With drugs, we can study the impact of two very controllable factors: the actual intervention, or the absence of the intervention. With nutritional interventions, this is not that easy. Why? On the continuum of nutritional status of a person, there are two extremes: complete deficiency and resultant death at one end, and toxicity from overdosage and resultant death at the other end. Most clinical trials examining a nutrient don't take into account whether a person is already deficient in that nutrient at the start of the study. Furthermore, trying to test a particular substance in a study does not account for the synergistic effects of a holistic lifestyle. In other words, in most cases, vitamins and herbs work best when used in combination with appropriate lifestyle modifications.

In the real world, if the intervention was applied to people who were deficient and needed the nutrient, the results would likely be positive. In a "controlled model," if the subjects were already above the threshold for the nutrient or compound, the results would more likely be negative. This is one of the main reasons that mixed results appear across clinical trials, and the "need for further study" is often mentioned.

Issue 6: The *effects* of nutritional balance are not taken into account when studying different clinical outcomes. If you take too much of one nutrient, a deficiency in another can result. For example, too much zinc depletes copper. Naturopathic doctors are trained to assess the body for deficiencies and use modalities that take into account the balancing of these effects. Clinical trials do not account for these interactions. They test the intervention, but not necessarily the appropriate use of it.

But ... Is Natural Medicine Really Safe?

Now, what about people who are concerned about the profile of safety for natural substances? That many people worry more about potential side effects of herbs than of pharmaceuticals is further evidence of the marketing of fear and money (versus an emphasis on healing from a truly unbiased stance). The potential for harm from natural substances is absolutely incomparable to the potential harm from conventional drugs.

A June 2013 review[13] published in *Medscape* reported only two deaths from vitamins, including overdose, out of 61,126 exposures:

> Morbidity and mortality from pure vitamins are rare ... [The] American Association of Poison Control Centers reported more than 61,000 single exposures to vitamins in 2011, but only 2 deaths resulted.[13]

The Centers for Disease Control and Prevention (CDC) even states the following about cardiovascular disease, the leading cause of death: "A healthy diet and lifestyle are the best weapons you have to fight heart disease. Many people make it harder than it is."[14] Meanwhile, various studies are arriving at the same conclusion. The INTERHEART study,[15] published in *The Lancet*, examined risk factors among 15,152 heart attack patients and 14,820 controls and drew the following conclusion regarding lifestyle and heart disease:

> Abnormal lipids, smoking, hypertension, diabetes, abdominal obesity, psychosocial factors, consumption of fruits, vegetables, and alcohol, and regular physical activity account for most of the risk of myocardial infarction worldwide in both sexes and at all ages in all regions. This finding suggests that approaches to

> *prevention can be based on similar principles worldwide and have the potential to prevent most premature cases of myocardial infarction.*[15]

The United States currently ranks 14th in overall mortality. *Fourteenth!* And that's with *half* of adults age 45 and older taking statins, which many doctors view as a wonder drug for the heart. Something's obviously missing in the health equation.

The old Hippocratic quote, "Let food be thy medicine, thy medicine shall be thy food," echoes in my head as I write this. Although it may seem too simple to use diet and lifestyle as a form of medicine, it is the oldest prescription around, dating back to the father of medicine. Now science is catching up with that wisdom.

We will talk more about food as a healing source throughout this book. For now, I ask you to open your mind to the not-so-terrific statistics of conventional medicine and to the robust healing possibilities of nature. Consider that everything you need to prevent and mitigate symptoms is not just behind the pharmacist's counter, but also accessible right at your fingertips.

CHAPTER 2

A New Approach to Individualized Treatment

I consider myself incredibly fortunate not only to be working in a field I love, but having the opportunity to work with each and every one of my clients. Every day, I am graced with miracles sitting in front of me, and the wonderment of that reality fuels my work. As a holistic doctor, my job is to help decode the messages from my clients' bodies, and to assist them in giving their bodies what they need to heal. I also seek to remove any obstacles that may be blocking this transformation. Then I get out of the way so that the client's *vis medicatrix naturae*, innate and vital life force, can do the rest.

Because every person is unique, with a specific physical and spiritual makeup, my role as doctor shifts with each one. Some clients need a coach to recommend only slight adjustments in their lifestyle; whereas, others need nutritional advice to change their diet or to add a few supplements to correct nutritional deficiencies. For others, the picture is more complex. There's more to the story, more labels attached to them over time, more thought patterns that have taken hold. Here's where my role as a doctor becomes coach, nutritionist, physician, detective, and biochemist. Nutritional intake, case history, blood work, clinical imaging, and functional tests serve as my guides in decoding the messages of the body. These tools allow me to view the body at the cellular level where function has often initially gone awry, and provide me with a means for correction.

In the last chapter, we talked about some of the scarier aspects of conventional medicine. As a naturopath, I am not against most of the modern techniques that Western medicine has to offer ... to the contrary! I am in awe, for instance, of the diagnostic systems at our fingertips, since they allow for a means of assessment that is necessary and illuminating (no pun intended). But what saddens me about conventional medicine today is that it's too busy trying to fix and manipulate systems. We confuse the alleviation of symptoms with true healing.

Shifting the Outlook on "Wellness"

So many of us have been programmed to view "treatment" as consisting of aggressive interventions, fighting against the body's determination to be sick. But let's take one step backward, to where illness *begins to take root*. The worrisome truth is that most people are too frightened to go here. We worry about our health, yet we don't want to change the habits or thought patterns that negatively affect our well-being. We hurriedly eat lunch while surfing through emails, medicate ourselves with uppers and downers, and head outside for a cigarette when the workday becomes too intense. We allow our bodies to be cut open as a means of healing, rather than viewing this as a last resort if our bodies aren't able to remove obstacles by themselves. In a sense, we view the body as an opponent that must be conquered!

When we start to *feel* unwell, we rush to spend our co-pays on doctors who can evaluate the symptoms that our bodies might be producing to call attention to a problem, and we silence the messages!

We have been trained to believe that every single ache and pain is wrong and that something must be done to make them disappear. Our hyperactive minds are no longer willing to sit still long enough to determine whether the issue at hand might be related to our lifestyles and a need to tweak them. Instead, we take a pill to diminish our physical symptoms as quickly as possible. This is understandable, for who wants to feel pain? The underlying cause, however, is ignored. As a result, the pains tend to return, and we pill-pop and doctor-hop, to whammy-whack every symptom that appears.

Dr. Mark Hyman, Chairman of the Institute for Functional Medicine, recipient of the 2009 Linus Pauling Award for Leadership in Functional Medicine, and medical editor at the *Huffington Post*, talks about the effects of treating symptoms over causes:

> *Just because you're treating your symptoms doesn't mean you're healthy. If you think your doctor is controlling your health problems because he or she has prescribed medication for them — well, you couldn't be more wrong!*
>
> *That's because doctors are very well trained to treat symptoms and diseases, but NOT to address the underlying imbalances that perpetuate illness.*[1]

The real solution to health issues is using an approach that identifies the root cause of imbalances in the body. This is partly accomplished by determining how your various symptoms might be connected to each other, not by looking at just one problem in isolation. This approach also focuses on balancing the interrelationship of every organ system, rather than focusing on only one body part. It is called "systems medicine" and moves beyond symptom relief and into the achievement of *optimal* health.

Searching for a Miracle Pill

Part of modern medicine is the search for the almighty pill that will keep us healthy, strong, and young, without having to change our lifestyle patterns. The problem with this approach is that we think we can continue living a less-than-healthy lifestyle. Sooner or later, though, we're going to have to pay the piper! Unfortunately, in this day and age, this attitude too often results in adhering to a regimen of prescription drugs instead of addressing the lifestyle choices that caused the imbalance in the first place.

A 2011 article[2] in the *Archives of Internal Medicine* reported that the use of prescription medications has become excessive. With the emergence of superbugs and the explosion of chronic diseases related to modifiable lifestyle factors, it's becoming apparent that now is the time to utilize another approach in medicine. The article offers six steps to deter the physician from over-prescribing the drug flavor of the month:

> *Judicious prescribing is a prerequisite for safe and appropriate medication use. Based on evidence and lessons from recent studies demonstrating problems with widely prescribed medications, we offer a series of principles as a prescription for more cautious and conservative prescribing. These principles urge clinicians to (1) think beyond drugs (consider nondrug therapy, treatable underlying causes, and prevention); (2) practice more strategic prescribing (defer nonurgent drug treatment; avoid unwarranted drug switching; be circumspect about unproven drug uses; and start treatment with only 1 new drug at a time); (3) maintain heightened vigilance regarding adverse effects (suspect drug reactions; be aware of withdrawal syndromes; and educate patients to anticipate reactions); (4) exercise caution and skepticism*

regarding new drugs (seek out unbiased information; wait until drugs have sufficient time on the market; be skeptical about surrogate rather than true clinical outcomes; avoid stretching indications; avoid seduction by elegant molecular pharmacology; beware of selective drug trial reporting); (5) work with patients for a shared agenda (do not automatically accede to drug requests; consider nonadherence before adding drugs to regimen; avoid restarting previously unsuccessful drug treatment; discontinue treatment with unneeded medications; and respect patients' reservations about drugs); and (6) consider long-term, broader impacts (weigh long-term outcomes, and recognize that improved systems may outweigh marginal benefits of new drugs).[2]

A More Individualized Approach to Medicine

Healthcare, in the truest sense, is not a one-size-fits-all pill or protocol. Unfortunately, our culture has been trained to believe that every human organism (over 7 billion of us!) fits the same exact mold when it comes to illness and healing. Hence, there exists the belief that every symptom calls for the same pill, or at least the same pill category.

The healthcare market is currently flooded with various categories of caregivers. The most familiar, perhaps, are medical doctors who typically have only minimal exposure to integrative medicine and natural treatments for health problems – internists, general practitioners, and the like. Another type of caregiver is the "health specialist," who may or may not be a doctor but who gets "certified" to use an alternative approach through self-certification courses that have little standardization and that are not usually endorsed by the federal government or a specific medical society. Indeed, they generally offer training in the prescribing of formulas and cookie-cutter protocols that are "more natural." However, the education provided at weekend seminars or long-distance programs do not replace the extensive education of a truly integrative physician who prescribes treatment based on the individual, not on a protocol prescribed for a certain type of symptom or diagnosis.

The problem is *not* that either of these groups is lacking in skills or ability, but that they are guiding patients with only half of the picture in mind. We cannot hope to accomplish a change in health outcomes by remaining in the mindset that symptoms need to be suppressed and fought, whether by drugs or herbs – the underlying cause will continue to be evaded. We need a systems-based medicine addressing individual needs. This can be achieved with the help of practitioners who use their diagnostic skills to treat the cause, versus technicians that use a protocol geared toward eradicating symptoms of a disease.

There is a saying in medicine: "when all you have is a hammer, everything looks like a nail." In other words, a practitioner tends to treat an illness according to the tools (diagnostic, philosophic) at his or her disposal, not necessarily based on what will facilitate true healing.

Naturopathic training takes a much broader view. To give you a better idea of its underlying philosophy, I have paraphrased the six guiding principles of naturopathic medicine:

Six Guiding Principles of Naturopathic Medicine[3]

1. **The Healing Power of Nature**
   Vis Medicatrix Naturae
   The body has an inborn ability to maintain and re-establish health. If the body becomes imbalanced, the process of restoring health is based on the natural order of life force that is innate in every individual. The physician should facilitate and work with this process through identification and removal of obstacles to health and to support a healthy internal and external environment.

2. **Identify and Treat the Cause**
   Tolle Causam
   Any illness has an underlying cause. In order for a body to fully heal, the physician should seek to find the cause by analyzing all of the symptoms within the context of the disease process. Symptoms should be viewed as the body's attempts to heal and should not automatically be suppressed. Once all underlying causes are identified, at the physical, emotional, and spiritual levels, a physician and patient may decide to suppress certain symptoms. But this is done by using the most non-invasive means possible. Once health is fully restored, symptoms are no longer expressed, and the additional support can be discontinued.

3. **First, Do No Harm**
   Primum No Nocere
   Disease and illness is a purposeful process that is aimed at restoring balance. Healing may include symptoms as part of the body's attempt to reestablish health. A physician should honor this process by supporting the viz medicatrix naturae in the least invasive means possible. Methods to eliminate symptoms, without addressing underlying causes, should be avoided or minimized, as they may well cause further harm.

4. **Treat the Whole Person**
   Tolle Totum
   The physician must consider the whole person when treating disease. This means that the complex interaction of physical, spiritual, mental, emotional, genetic, environmental, social, and other factors should be evaluated when restoring health. Evaluating all factors is essential to fully recover from disease and to aid in prevention of future illness.

5. **The Physician as Teacher**
   Docere
   The physician's relationship with the patient is as important as the correct diagnosis and appropriate prescription. This therapeutic relationship has healing powers of its own inherent value. The physician should educate the patient in how to be accountable for their own healing. The physician must strive to be an example of health and continue to develop his/her own personal and spiritual development as a teacher.

6. **Prevention is the Best "Cure"**
   Through education and promotion of healthy lifestyle habits, the physician should aim at preventing future diseases. This is the ultimate goal of any healthcare system. Therefore, once health is restored, the physician should establish genetic susceptibility and risk factors that could be risk for future illness. Emphasis should be placed on empowering the patient to avoid unhealthy actions and promote health, rather than fight disease.

Although a conventional physician may embrace some of the concepts mentioned above, he will probably not incorporate the whole picture in a 15-minute visit. For example, an internist may mention lifestyle factors to a patient with diabetes, such as exercise and dietary changes. Most likely, however, he or she will not provide a comprehensive, individualized treatment approach that includes diet, coaching, nutritional, and lifestyle support to guide the process along. A naturopathic or functional medicine practitioner will fill in the gap between standard of care and personalized medicine.

Biochemistry: Honoring Your Unique Makeup

There exists a belief in integrative medicine that we are all much more than our bodies. We have yet to tap into our full understanding of the ancient energy system that is now being discussed and explained by the laws of physics. Still, we are subject to the physical laws of biochemistry, which keep us bound to balancing certain elements within the body for optimum health. The balance of these constituents exists in different mixtures and ratios in different individuals.

For example, did you ever wonder why a particular treatment works wonders for one person, but causes harm in another, despite the fact that the same exact dosage or brand is used? This is the concept of *biochemical individuality*, first introduced by noted biochemist Roger Williams, PhD, in his 1952 work, *A Physician's Handbook on Orthomolecular Medicine*. Williams presents a cohesive genotropic theory of diseases: "The biological capabilities of a person are set by his/her genotype; these interact with the environment (which includes the nutritional milieu of the cell as well as the external physical, emotional, and social environment) to produce the phenotype of the individual, and the diseases to which he is susceptible."

According to nutritional biochemist and researcher, Alexander Schauss,

> The genetotropic principal states, "Every individual organism has a distinctive genetic background and distinctive nutrition needs that must be met for optimal wellbeing." To disregard this principal and simply rely

> upon a committee's recommendation for a nutrient that has been determined to play such an important role in human health is nothing short of disregarding the individual needs of the patient.[4]

Individualized biochemistry opens up an interesting dialogue in healthcare. Just as we should not reach for a single "miracle pill" to make everything better, we should not put all of our faith into one nutrient. This is because everyone has a different genetic makeup, and one that interacts with unique lifestyle patterns and dietary components. Different stressors, diets, and lifestyle factors create different imbalances in different individuals.

This fact alone makes ONE miracle vitamin, supplement, or herb an *impossibility*! Let's take Vitamin D as an example. It has been hypothesized, that in a person with autoimmune disease such as lupus or autoimmune thyroid disease, Vitamin D supplementation might actually exacerbate the hyperactive immune response.[5] On the other hand, in someone with breast cancer, it could be the missing nutrient to signal the receptor sites to turn on apoptosis, the body's natural method for destroying damaged cells.

Furthermore, just as side effects from medications differ between different people, side effects from nutrients can occur in different people for different reasons. For this reason, I get nervous when I hear of anyone self-prescribing to treat symptoms. This is especially scary when decisions are based on a single article or the advice of a medical "expert" proclaiming the benefits of a particular nutrient in which the seller has a financial investment.

The takeaway from this is clear: toying with biochemistry is a serious issue, and not something to be done without professional guidance. It's like tinkering with your car without any knowledge of mechanics. Most people wouldn't dream of fixing a broken-down vehicle by just throwing a highly-touted engine degreaser under the hood and getting back behind the wheel without checking to see how the other parts were affected! What if the degreaser is irrelevant to your engine's problem? What will happen to your car 10, 20, 30 miles down the road?

Overloading on a particular nutrient or supplement without knowing its effects can turn into a game of supplement roulette with one's biochemistry. At best, a symptom is suppressed without treating the cause (which means that you can expect more symptoms in the future). At worst, serious interactions occur, depleting the body of other nutrients, and creating more issues.

All Systems Go ... Together

One of the strongest precepts of functional medicine and naturopathy is that every system in your body affects the other systems. This may not seem like an earth-shattering revelation at first, but did you know, for example, that an imbalance of your hormones can affect your digestion? Or that your spiritual well-being can affect your brain's neurotransmitters? Or that your activity level can affect the amount of inflammation in your body?

What you ingest can have far-reaching, unintended effects as well. What happens when someone has a plethora of symptoms and is taking several medications along with many supplements? What interactions exist between one medication and just a few supplements? Even the most highly sought-after and well-known integrative doctors will tell you that the answers are, as yet, inconclusive. Dr. Leo Galland, a well-known functional medicine expert, discusses the complicated interactions of herbs, drugs, and nutrients in his seminar on Nutrient-Drug Interactions, through the Institute of Functional Medicine.[6] Here are a few examples:

1. The supplement curcumin, a constituent found in the Indian spice, turmeric, can have anti-inflammatory synergism with resveratrol; but can be antagonized when taken with another

supplement, N-acetylcysteine (NAC). It also has a complicated dose response with green tea.
2. Vitamin E and statins are not a good mix. Furthermore, vitamin E, in the form of alpha-tocopherol, reduces coenzyme Q10 (CoQ10), a nutrient vital for heart health. However, when the whole form of vitamin E is used (i.e., mixed tocopherols), or other components of this vitamin (tocotrienols), a different response is mediated.
3. St. John's wort can stimulate the liver detoxification pathway, CYP3A4, resulting in decreased blood levels of many medications. It can also act as a dose-dependent inhibitor or stimulator of intestinal drug clearance via P-gp. This results in drug interactions with 50 percent of medications cleared by these liver pathways.

The study of systems biology and functional medicine, along with the naturopathic philosophy of treating the specific cause of a disease, provides a biochemical, genetic, and systematic framework that is tailored to each individual. Philosophy, science, and mind-body medicine unite in a perfect balance of these comprehensive trainings as they are applied on an individualized basis.

Looking Forward

My mentors inspire me every day to read more, learn more, and keep up with the current research and ancient wisdom, all the while keeping my focus on the uniqueness of the individual client. This helps me distinguish which sexy nutrient of the moment is helpful, hurtful, or hype, based on each individual's unique needs.

My first task when working with my clients is to determine their specific needs. We then compile the best plan for them based on what their body's specific nutrient needs, health history, lifestyle factors, and current diagnostics show us. Integration is truly the key to the best possible assessment and treatment. We combine the diagnostic skills of conventional medicine with the biochemistry of nutrients and medicine for a beautiful synergism in healthcare and prevention!

Here's an example of how this model provided a solution to one of my client's struggles to find answers for her uncomfortable bladder and gastrointestinal discomfort. Colleen writes:

> *Dr. Sarah, you have been a God-send! After a few months of really uncomfortable bladder and stomach issues that interfered with daily activities, I was ready to give up. Practitioners of conventional medicine suggested that my bladder probably "just doesn't work right" and more than likely would have put me on medication to mask my symptoms without getting to the root of the problem. That didn't sit right with me.*
>
> *That's when I started to explore natural and holistic medicine. That's when I met you. During my first appointment, I had your undivided attention for well over an hour. You delved into my family history, my medical history, my mental and emotional health, as well as asked pertinent questions regarding my symptoms. You took down pages of notes and I felt like you really listened to me and aimed to treat me as a whole person, not just my symptoms. I felt like you cared. You were able to pin-point the root of the problem in that very first visit and prescribed a change in diet and a regimen of natural supplements. I left your office feeling hope for the first time in months!*
>
> *I have been a patient for not quite a year now and am a completely different (and much healthier) person than when I first walked into your office. Over the last several months, you worked with me and my nutritionist*

> *to figure out what type of nutritional regimen and whole food supplements work for me. No medication! I hope to be your patient for a very long time ... I recommend you to everyone!*

In this scenario, the diagnostics of Colleen's primary care doctors and specialists were integrated into the best treatment plan for her. Medications were not benefiting Colleen, so we explored the results she could obtain from a comprehensive and more natural program. For Colleen, this meant lifestyle and dietary adjustments, nutritional supplementation, and mind-body techniques.

CHAPTER 3

Let Food Be Thy Medicine

Confucius is credited with saying, "To do good work, one must have good tools." The best tool to start with for optimum physical and emotional health is a healthy diet. However, as a society, we simply eat far too much junk. And just as drugs alter our body chemistry, so do the foods we eat. Therefore, it's safe to assume that our diet will affect our total health. As an overall concept, we refer to this as *nutrigenomics*, or the ways in which the foods we eat affect how our DNA – our genetic material – is read. This, in turn, can affect the way in which foods are absorbed, transported, and used in the body. And *this*, in turn, affects every single system in the body!

In a culture where we are sent mixed messages to eat healthfully yet enter grocery stores filled with sugar-laden temptations, it becomes a battle for most people to tune into their bodies' true needs. Furthermore, many of the foods available to us in the grocery store have been developed by chemists, not nutritionists. Tinkering with natural food sources has resulted in longer shelf-life and greater convenience, but the "food" is often devoid of essential nutrients and phytochemicals. Instead, preservatives, harmful fillers, additives, colorings, sugar, and/or artificial sweeteners are added. These chemicals not only cause nutrient depletion, but also result in addiction from the effects they can have on satiety (hunger signals), absorption, and digestive cues in the body.

So, to whom can we turn for the right information? Probably not to the media or one-size-fits-all books published by "celebrity experts." It's up to each of us to become educated consumers. From this vantage point, we can then identify the true health experts and which choices are best for our own biochemistry.

Start with a Positive Outlook

Every day, I hear stories from various clients about how they are monitoring everything that goes into their mouths, working out harder, cutting out more calories, avoiding food allergens, and yet are gaining weight! Depressed from the lack of results after "doing everything right," they invariably enter into a cycle of restrictive-binge eating patterns. These cycles cause their brain's thermostat for weight maintenance and brain chemistry to become dysregulated and to misfire. The result is a vicious, self-perpetuating cycle into what I call the "grumpy dieter's deprivation blues."

I've found that these dieters are usually obsessively preoccupied with their image; they're overweight, angry, and self-deprecating. Their very life existence is based on a bookmark somewhere between being fat and miserable and being thin and, therefore, happy. Not a fun space to be in! Many believe that this negative self-talk will motivate them to change eating behaviors; however, this is usually not the case. In fact, science is showing us that people who have a more positive self-image are actually thinner to begin with. As a result, they tend to be more self-compassionate and have less dysfunctional eating behavioral patterns.

Recently, I came across an article in the *Vital Choice* newsletter that discussed the findings from a study linking self-compassion with healthy behaviors, including eating.[1] Similar studies support this concept, linking changes in brain biochemistry to unhealthy eating behavior. Specifically, there exists a paradox of binge eating following restriction, with resultant weight gain. According to the article, researchers found that men and women with a more self-accepting attitude had less restrictive eating patterns, more self-acceptance, and better overall health. In fact, the non-restrictors ended up eating less than the restrictors in the long run!

Intrigued, I found the original study posted in the *Journal of Social and Clinical Psychology*.[2] The study investigated whether self-compassion would alleviate the common unhealthy behavior in food restrictors to overeat after eating unhealthy foods. The study focused on college women who completed measures of rigid and restrained eating, restrictive eating, and feeling guilty after eating unhealthy foods. The participants were then asked to either eat or not eat an unhealthy food and were instructed to think self-compassionately and without judgment following their decision. The results indicated that self-compassion reduced distress and did, in fact, prevent eating the unhealthy food in restrictive eaters.

This study demonstrated that positive feelings could trump stress-producing hormones that create inflammation and resultant weight gain. In other words, the more stressed-out you are about what you eat, the more likely you'll make poor food choices and the less likely you'll enjoy life. To spin it in a positive way, enjoy what you eat and you'll weigh less!

Other investigators had this to say about the power of self-compassion:

> *Feelings of compassion for self and others have been linked to higher levels of brain activation in the left prefrontal cortex, a region associated with joy and optimism. Results indicated that self-compassionate individuals experienced significantly more positive and less negative mood generally...*

> *Although self-compassion is associated with positive affect, it stems from the ability to hold difficult negative emotions in non-judgmental awareness without denial or suppression.*[3]

Biochemical Imbalances Result in Cravings

It's important to note that it's easier said than done for some people to stop consuming foods that don't replenish the body. Food addiction is a very real and serious issue in this day and age. Chemicals in modern food that were never intended to be used in our bodies can cause great harm on many levels. Some are seen and felt readily, while others take hold more slowly.

Mark Hyman, MD, makes the following points to describe similarities between food substances and drugs:[4]

1. The same neurotransmitter (dopamine) that stimulates the brain's reward center with drug use is also stimulated by sugar.
2. Ingestion of sugar and fat-laden foods produces a similar brain-imaging pattern (PET scan) as that produced by heroin, opium, or morphine, and stimulates the body to release its own opioids, which are a natural form of morphine.
3. Lower dopamine receptors in obese individuals (as illustrated by brain-imaging patterns) resemble those of drug addicts, and are thought to make them crave more addictive substances to compensate.
4. Naltrexone, which is used to block the brain receptors for heroin and morphine, reduces the consumption of high-sugar and high-fat foods.
5. People (and rodents) develop tolerance to sugar, similar to a drug addict, causing them to increase their intake to feel satisfied.

6. Despite negative social, health, and personal consequences, obese individuals tend to continue to eat unhealthy food substances, similar to an addict.
7. Dependency on a food continues past the state of enjoyment, to the point of eating simply to feel normal, similar to what happens in drug addiction.

If solving food addiction was a simple matter of education, i.e., understanding that junk food is bad for you, many would be able to stop; however, addictions tend to cloud our sense of reason and encourage rationalizations that perpetuate a harmful behavior, despite an obvious connection between the behavior and chronic symptoms.

Food sensitivities and allergies biochemically alter our ability to choose wisely. They can act on the reward system of the brain, producing insatiable cravings and excessive consumption. Therefore, it's not that people don't already suspect that their symptoms are connected to food; it's more that their brains can't handle the thought of existing without that dopamine surge!

The good news is that when the body is balanced, it doesn't need a dopamine surge to feel okay. People with food addictions do have natural support options to assist their bodies in achieving a balance that modulates their cravings. As an integrative doctor, it's important for me to look equally at the emotional and physical imbalances in the body that are contributing to cravings for a specific food that it never can get "enough" of.

Easing Into Healthy Food Choices: Balancing the Body

It's true that we are what we eat *and* what we absorb. If your digestive tract isn't absorbing food due to improper cues, quantities, or food sensitivities, the gut-brain connection goes awry. Physically balancing these cues and signals is important for toning down inflammation and tuning up absorption. This is done by assessing and treating nutritional deficiencies, neurotransmitter imbalances, hormonal and blood sugar dysregulation, and imbalanced gut microflora.

If all of these factors are fully addressed, then optimal absorption, assimilation, and biochemistry is obtained. Supporting all of these key players can actually aid or break an addictive, unhealthy relationship with food. Furthermore, when we are functioning at our body's full potential, we are truly more able to hear and trust our own hunger signals. Unfortunately, years of chronic dieting and the consumption of chemical-laden foods have left many people out of touch with their true appetites.

Tuning In

According to famous gastroenterologist and bariatric surgeon Dr. Michael Snyder, the biology of hunger and satiety is influenced by a combination of structural, biochemical, and behavioral feedback loops. As he states in his book, *The Full Diet*,[5]

> [The "cardia"] is where a legion of stretch receptors reacts to food physically filling your stomach ... It takes about 20-30 minutes after you start eating for the crescendo effect of ... your appetite hormones [e.g., leptin, ghrelin, peptide YY] to hit the conscious part of you that acknowledges you're full ... If we are not mindful of this effect, we can eat through any reasonable sense of fullness of this effect.[5]

When we eat real foods, which provide accurate signaling and secretion of these hunger-satiety molecules in our body, knowing when we're full is a lot easier.

Recently, one of my clients explained how she achieved a healthier weight by focusing on health and happiness rather than by worrying about calories and exercising like crazy. I encouraged her through our time together to focus less on counting, and more on nourishing her body. We implemented this with a specific, anti-inflammatory, whole foods diet along with a movement and nutritional program tailored to her unique biochemical needs.

The result was not just weight loss; Maggie was able to achieve a happier, healthier brain and body! She was shocked and pleased at her revived ability to feel her body's cues again and act accordingly. She lost 15 pounds and became pregnant (a personal goal). Maggie's self-care and dedication to her own nourishment had profound effects not just for her, but for her whole family.

Maggie is a testimony to the concept that the more we reconnect to our own natural state of well-being and seek professional guidance to rebalance our biochemistry, the more we are returned to a state of health, with less struggle and more joy. Go figure!

Your Perfect Diet: Embrace Your Individuality!

The subject of nutrition seems to be packed with a lot of heated controversy among experts. Dietary advice ranges from raw-food-vegetarianism to a cavemen diet of meat and vegetables. What to do?? By now you have probably already guessed my answer – it depends on the person!

As mentioned previously, the diet that is best for any individual has little to do with calorie counting and perfect proportion control. Rather, optimal choices in nutrition have more to do with individual lifestyle patterns, biochemical and genetic differences, blood type, ethnicity, current health status, and other physiological issues. Various combinations of foods affect our biology, not just by causing weight gain or weight loss, but by modifying our blood sugar, hormones, neurotransmitters, and brain health. The phytochemicals present in foods have the capacity to act as a medicine or a poison, with the effect varying from person to person.

Dr. Daniel Amen highlights this concept of different foods for different people relating to a person's mindset.[6] Dr. Amen's approach to dietary suggestions is found by focusing on individual variations in brain types. For example, those who have compulsive eating patterns are guided to add some much-villainized carbohydrates into their diet. This type of eater tends to grab, obsess, and fantasize about a certain food until it is finally consumed. Healthy carbohydrates (complex carbohydrates such as whole grains, beans and legumes) help replete compulsive eaters' low brain serotonin levels. Furthermore, eating healthy carbohydrates allows the amino acid that becomes this neurotransmitter to more easily cross the blood-brain barrier, thereby calming an overanxious and compulsive eater.

On the other hand, more impulsive folks already have enough serotonin. These unbalanced eaters tend to grab a "treat" they know isn't good for them, simply because of its proximity or environmental cues. With impulsive eaters, increasing brain dopamine is often helpful. Eating fewer carbohydrates and healthier proteins such as organic meats, fish, and nuts and seeds protects the body from sugar rushes and satiates the increased need for dopamine. Some people are compulsive-impulsive overeaters (combination of the two), in which case eating equal ratios of carbohydrates and proteins is recommended.

In the above scenarios, picture an impulsive person on a vegetarian diet (mostly carbohydrate) or a compulsive person on a cavemen diet (mostly protein), each simply following the latest diet craze. Their weight may even out, but will their brain and hormones? Add into this picture the potential of inflammatory processes, digestive impairment, food sensitivities, and heart disease. A-one-diet-for-all just doesn't make sense!

Pass Up the Gluten

I'm not a big fan of generalizations, but there are some classes of foods I recommend that most of my clients avoid or at least eat less of. This is because these foods lack nutritional value or may actually cause harm. I believe common sensitivities to these foods are more due to food overproduction and processing by the food industry than to the actual food itself. One such food class is gluten (a protein in grains such as wheat, barley, and rye).

Unfortunately, symptomatic reactions to gluten are becoming more and more evident. According to Dr. Christiane Northrup,[7] one of the reasons so many people are so sensitive to gluten today is because wheat bread has been manufactured to have ten times the amount of protein content than if produced in its natural state. This is in order to increase the fluff, market value, and taste of bread. Our bodies just aren't designed to digest that kind of protein profile. (It has even been suggested that, in Europe, where genetically-modified ingredients and mass devaluing of grains was a lot less prevalent, there existed less grain sensitivity).

Part of my job as an integrative doctor is to teach a person that digestive health is not just measured by gastrointestinal distress. Not feeling bloated, gassy, or suffering from loose stools after eating a certain food doesn't mean that the food you're eating is optimal for your whole system.

Your digestive tract is responsible for more than just absorption and digestion; it's also the home of an intricate regulation between absorption, elimination, immune function, and brain health. In fact, it has its own unique immune and nervous systems – the GALT (gut-associated lymphoid tissue) and the ENS (enteric nervous system). What you put in your mouth influences the health of your immune system, nervous system, hormones, brain, and overall body processes.

The possible negative effects of gluten consumption in people who are sensitive to it are diverse, ranging from anxiety and thyroid imbalances, to inflammation and immune issues. Many people who have heard of celiac disease assume that it's a gluten allergy. Celiac disease, however, is an autoimmune disorder, in which the immune system attacks the lining of the small intestine as it attacks gluten; an intestinal biopsy is required to confirm the diagnosis. This is very different from an allergic reaction, in which the immune system mounts an IgE antibody reaction to a substance (usually involving histamine release) but doesn't attack the body's own tissues. Autoimmune disorders only occur in people who are genetically predisposed to them.

It appears that gluten reactions can be autoimmune (including celiac disease, but also in parts of the body outside the intestine), allergic (usually a wheat allergy), or in a category all by itself (neither immune- or autoimmune-mediated, but still causing symptoms). Certain antibodies can be measured in the lab – tTG (anti-tissue transglutaminase) and EMA (anti-endomysial antibody) – that are specific for celiac disease. In contrast, AGAs (anti-gliadin antibodies) suggest an immune reaction to gluten, but don't necessarily point to intestinal celiac disease. A study published in the *Journal of Scandinavia Gastroenterology*[8] supports this idea, and also suggested a specific brain-gut and gut-joint connection for gluten:

> *Although AGA positivity is of clinical relevance only in a subset of elderly people, it seems to be related to rheumatoid arthritis and depression, both conditions linked to celiac disease. Further studies are needed to reveal the mechanisms underlying this. The poor specificity of AGA for celiac disease was here once more in evidence.*[8]

The clinical implications of this study are astounding, and are already familiar to most naturopathic doctors. Treating the gut is not only about digestion, but also about treating the brain and whole body! Various research studies have shown that sensitivity to wheat can be linked to autoimmune conditions other than celiac in some individuals, and may be a marker for other chronic diseases down the line.

Dr. Aristo Vojdani describes how increased permeability in our gut lining, or "leaky gut," can play a big role in systemic and chronic diseases through the following pathway:[9]

> Mucosal immune abnormalities →
> Imbalanced gut flora (big players in your immune system) →
> Induction of intestinal barrier dysfunction →
> Release of inflammatory mediators into circulation →
> Enhanced systemic inflammation and damage to tissues →
> Open blood-brain barrier, resulting in neuroinflammation →
> Neuro-invasion and neurodegeneration

This is not just a theory. According to the Academy of Science,[10] wheat enteropathy can be linked to chronic disease, specifically multiple sclerosis. Researchers studied 98 patients with multiple sclerosis and were able to determine the level of serum IgA and IgG anti-gliadin (AGAs) and anti-tissue transglutaminase antibodies (anti-tTGs), which are specific immune markers of gluten. They reported,

> We found a highly significant increase in titers of immunoglobulin G antibodies against gliadin and tissue transglutaminase in the multiple sclerosis patients. Seven patients had a positive IgG AGA, whereas only 2 controls presented positive titers ($P = 0.03$). Four patients had positive IgG anti-tTG while all the controls tested negative ($P = 0.02$).

I check for gluten reactions in the majority of my clients through a combination of a gluten-elimination diet (and watching for changes in symptoms) and celiac blood panels in which I track the levels of the abovementioned antibodies to gluten. Even if the number of antibodies isn't high enough to suggest celiac disease, elevated antibodies still indicate an immune reaction to gluten in one's system.

I explain these findings to my clients in the following way: "whether the label of 'celiac disease' applies or not, your body is making antibodies against a food. This causes your immune system to be over-stimulated and to produce a specific immune response in the body. This would not happen if this substance was deemed 'harmless.'"

What About Wheat in Another Form?

Many people believe that *sprouted* wheat may not have the same effect on the body's immune system. Clinically, I have not found this to be true, thus unfortunately cannot recommend sprouted wheat as a good alternative.

Dr. Joseph Mercola, an osteopathic physician, leading health expert, and founder of one of the top natural health websites,[11] summarized the problems with a wheat-containing glycoprotein (called "wheat germ agglutinin, or WGA"), responsible for adverse effects in the body, including immune (autoimmunity, cytotoxicity), inflammatory, digestive, brain (excitotoxicity and neurotoxicity), heart, and endocrine (thyroid):

> Interestingly enough, the highest amounts of WGA are found in whole wheat, including its sprouted form, which is touted as being the most healthful form of all. Aside from high amounts of WGA, wheat also contains a number of other potentially health-harming components, including:
> - Gliadin (an alcohol-soluble protein component)
> - Gliadomorphins (exorphins, or group of opioid molecules that form during digestion of the gluten protein)
> - Enzyme inhibitors

Rye and barley are included in this WGA family as well. Dr. Mercola also suggested that both potato and tomato may contain similar reactive lectins, specifically chitin lectins, which may cause the identical negative health reactions as wheat.

The Benefits of a Gluten-Free Mood

As described above, the gut and brain are intricately connected. A recent study,[12] featured in *Biological Psychology*, demonstrated the harmful effects of gluten reactions on brain health by correlating lab markers to gluten sensitivity in patients with schizophrenia or recent-onset psychosis. The investigators concluded,

> *Individuals with recent-onset psychosis and with multi-episode schizophrenia who have increased antibodies to gliadin may share some immunologic features of celiac disease, but their immune response to gliadin differs from that of celiac disease.*[12]

Which brings me back to my point ... Could the rise in chronic diseases and mood imbalances be ameliorated by changing what we're feeding our bodies, rather than by popping pills into our mouths to suppress the symptoms?

Another article in the same journal reported over 20 years ago that this may indeed be the case:

> *If, as hypothesized, neuroactive peptides from grain glutens are the major agents evoking schizophrenia in those with the genotype(s), it should be rare if grain is rare...*
>
> *When these peoples became partially westernized and consumed wheat, barley beer, and rice, the prevalence reached European levels. Our findings agree with previous*

> *epidemiologic and experimental results indicating that grain glutens are harmful to schizophrenics.*[13]

I have seen this gluten-symptom connection time and again. For example, I had one client who had depression, anxiety, and knee pain. Over the course of several months, she followed a comprehensive plan consisting of eliminating gluten, adding supportive nutrients for digestive health, and restoring her body's low stores of magnesium. She also was tested for a specific genetic marker, the methylene tetrahydrofolate reductase (MTHFR) gene. This gene effects how the body converts folate and folic acid and is intricately related to the methylation cycle. This cycle is important for many processes in the body including immune and cardiovascular health, detoxification, and neurotransmitter formation. This makes finding variances in this gene important for many reasons.

After three months, her anxiety was less, and after six months it had completely disappeared. Her depression and low mood were also improved, her joint pain went away, and she lost five pounds!

Dr. Hyman reported in a recent article[14] that hidden inflammation in the form of food sensitivities could be one of the root causes of chronic diseases such as depression, autoimmune disease, and heart disease. He reports on how addressing this issue helped one of his patients:

> *Food allergies cause inflammation, and studies now show inflammation in the brains of depressed people. In fact, researchers are studying powerful anti-inflammatory drugs used in autoimmune disease such as Enbrel for the treatment of depression.*
>
> *After she eliminated her IgG or delayed food allergies, her depression went away, she got off her medication — and she lost 30 pounds as a side effect!*[14]

Furthermore, in one study,[15] high levels of two markers of inflammation, C-reactive protein (CRP) and interleukin-6 (IL-6), in generally "healthy" elderly subjects were associated with a 260 percent increased risk of dying within the next four years, compared to those with lower levels of inflammation. Among the causes of death was cardiovascular disease, the risk of which we know is greatly influenced by lifestyle factors, including diet.

This effect is seen in our little ones as well. I have heard countless mothers comment on how different their "hyperactive and depressed child" now acts after removing certain foods that were identified as triggers. Recently, four-year-old Kevin's mom reported,

> *Dr. Sarah, he's a completely different person. He is calm and polite now. He is getting along with his classmates and his teachers report he appears more focused! Since we changed his diet and he's been consistently taking his supplements, it's been amazing and worth every penny!*

This example of Kevin provides evidence that these kids are not suffering from a Ritalin deficiency, but rather an imbalanced biochemistry. In Kevin's case, the root cause of mood and behavioral problems were food sensitivities that caused brain inflammation.

How to Go Gluten-Free

Use baby steps to make this dietary change. I recommend starting with breakfast and then eventually making all three meals consist of organic, whole, gluten-free foods. This could be one of the most powerful steps in transforming your overall health! See if you notice a difference within three weeks. Are your joints less achy? Is your mind clearer? Are you sleeping better?

If you're not sure at this point, reintroduce this protein-filled grain for one day, wait, and see how you respond after three days.

Sensitivities to foods are often delayed, causing various symptoms to occur between day one and three. For example, your skin could get itchy, eczema could flare, your mood could feel heavier, your joints creakier, and your sleep more disturbed. If these or any other symptoms appear, you may want to consider passing up gluten. (We will get more into gluten and leaky gut in Chapter 5).

The Sweetness of Life? Reconsidering Sugar

According to an article in *Psychology Today*, sugar can have effects on the brain that are similar to those of gluten:

> *First, sugar actually suppresses activity of a key growth hormone in the brain called BDNF. This hormone promotes the health and maintenance of neurons in the brain, and it plays a vital role in memory function by triggering the growth of new connections between neurons. BDNF levels are critically low in both depression and schizophrenia, which explains why both syndromes often lead to shrinkage of key brain regions over time (yes, chronic depression actually leads to brain damage).*[16]

The article also reports evidence from animal models that sugar can trigger inflammation. In the short term, inflammation can be a healing response, but in the long term can negatively affect activity in the brain and create havoc in immune functioning. In fact, chronic inflammation has been associated with increased risk of heart disease, diabetes, and other disease processes.

My clients are aware of my belief that biochemistry will trump willpower every time. So, if giving up gluten and sugar, even at one meal, is too difficult, there may be more to blame than just a food sensitivity.

In these cases, I will look for factors such as an underlying dysbiosis (imbalanced microflora in the gastrointestinal tract), neurotransmitter and hormonal imbalances, or a chronic blood sugar issue.

Strong emotions can surface when releasing physical dependencies on certain harmful foods. In fact, I've literally seen women cry when I've suggested giving up their coffee or cake. This is because, as mentioned, these foods can be addictive to the brain and body. Some may use them as an addict would use a drug, to numb emotional pain.

Therefore, I've found it imperative to provide my clients with social support tools that will assist them in eliminating their "comfort foods." In these instances, clients need more than just a list of "good" foods and "bad" foods. They need compassion and a support system to deal with the underlying reasons for eating those foods that they know are harming them.

The Case for and Against Soy

In a feature article on soy,[17] Dr. Mercola discussed the history of soy, from superhero to villain. He talked about how soy was introduced in the early 1990s as a natural miracle food. It was touted to lower cholesterol, aid in hot flashes, and protect against breast and prostate cancer.

Dr. Mercola's viewpoint is that most of these claims have been false and that the health-promoting aspects of soy are mostly used as a marketing ploy to promote soy as a healthy vegetarian alternative for protein. As a result, he advises consumers to avoid soy and find other healthy options. Furthermore, the fact that most of soy is genetically modified is an additional health risk for many.

So, are you convinced now that soy should completely be avoided? Not so fast; let's take another look. The Agency for HealthCare Research and Quality (AHRQ) wrote an unbiased, scientific, 245-page "summary" titled *The Effects of Soy on Health Outcomes*.[18] I'll save you the time to read it. Their main conclusion was that both the benefits and the harms of soy are probably overstated.

The effect of soy on women's health has been debated heavily. It seems that there exists a complex interaction between soy and estrogen, which may account for its harmful or healing effects in different women with different hormonal levels. According to authors of this same article,

> *Twelve studies reported estradiol levels at the follicular phase in 434 pre-menopausal women. The overall effect of soy on estradiol levels was not consistent. Most of the studies showed a trend for soy to reduce estradiol, although they failed to demonstrate a statistically significant effect.*[18]

Furthermore, the article reported that in six randomized trials reporting the effect of soy on thyroid-stimulating hormone (TSH), no overall effect of soy on TSH and thyroid function was clear.

Soy can act as an estrogen-mimic or an estrogen antagonist. For women who are low in estrogen, soy isoflavones (compounds in soy with weak estrogen-like actions) may actually be helpful. For women with estrogen-dominant patterns, high isoflavones may exacerbate symptoms or, if in their correct form, could block inflammatory estrogens at the cellular receptor site. Another factor to consider with regard to soy is the health of a woman's gastrointestinal tract. This will affect how well her intestinal bacteria can produce the beneficial compound, equol, from soy compounds. These various factors make it impossible to simply label soy as "good" or "bad," and may explain why there are such differing recommendations among brilliant doctors in the field.

In an interview[19] between Dr. Mercola and Dr. Christine Horner, a board certified general and plastic surgeon, Dr. Horner proposed that the explanation for these paradoxical effects could be attributed to foods' synergistic and modulating effects. Discussing this in relation to flax seeds, she explained how many different forms of estrogens exist, with different strengths and effects on the body. Estradiol is the strongest form; when it attaches to an estrogen receptor, it causes 1,000 cell divisions. Plant estrogens, on the other hand may cause only one division. Furthermore, if the body is flooded with plant estrogens, they can act to block stronger estrogens from attaching to its finite number of receptors, thus producing an inhibitory effect.

For children, soy in infant formula may interfere with hormonal regulation:

> *In 1998, investigators reported that the daily exposure of infants to isoflavones in soy infant formula is 6 to 11 times higher on a body-weight basis than the dose that has hormonal effects in adults consuming soy foods. Circulating concentrations of isoflavones in infants fed soy-based formula were 13,000 to 22,000 times higher than plasma estradiol concentrations in infants on cow's milk formula.*[20]

Dr. Mercola believes, therefore, that soy could have an impact on a variety of health conditions in children. These include: behavioral problems, digestive issues, hormonal and thyroid imbalances, early onset puberty or gynecomastia (female characteristics in males), and even cancer.

So what's the final word on soy? Good or bad? Superfood or fraud?

I do concur that fermented and non-GMO (non-genetically modified organism) soy products are the way to go. Non-organic soy contains aluminum, GMOs, pesticides, hormone mimics, and many harmful chemicals due to processing. This puts it back into the hands of very educated consumers or practitioners to know these important factors in order to determine whether soy will offer them the highest benefit.

And Then We Have the Super-Supplements...

Naturopathic and functional medicine doctors generally do not advocate for any one supplement, no matter how much great press it's currently receiving ... and for good reason. Vitamin D, for example, has recently found a place in the spotlight as one of the new super-supplements. By no means am I suggesting that vitamin D experts are not in touch with sound, valid research. I do believe that many of us are deficient in vitamin D and, as with any vitamin, we can expect positive results if we take it when we need it.

What I *am* saying is that unless we address the underlying issue of *why* a person is low in vitamin D in the first place, we might not get the results we want. This is because across-the-board recommendations without looking at causes of deficiencies or personal biochemistry can be dangerous. In the case of vitamin D, the impact of taking a fat-soluble vitamin in heavy doses by those with less efficient livers and kidneys – key players in the utilization of vitamin D – should be considered.

In a seminar on the subject of vitamin D, Dr. Alan Gaby expressed several concerns about high-dose vitamin D supplementation.[21] One of his concerns is that the majority of testing for vitamin D levels consists of measuring only one of its 50 monomers. This will not accurately reflect the total vitamin D concentration in an individual. Furthermore, he states that the beneficial effects of vitamin D have been based mostly on epidemiological studies. This means that high doses are associated with, but not necessarily the cause of, health benefits. In fact, until recently, few studies existed that demonstrated long-term safety of high-dose vitamin D supplementation to modulate health outcomes. Today, they are still sparse. Will vitamin D eventually be cast as a harmful supplement to be avoided at all costs in order to prevent possible overdosing? It's not unheard of for a vitamin to be exonerated one minute and villainized the next.

It seems that a nutrient is considered "bad" when it doesn't produce one straightforward biochemical effect on every single person who consumes it. Using generalizations based on epidemical studies have many stumbling blocks (see Chapter 1). Nutrients aren't drugs, and there isn't one supplement that can act as a Band-Aid for everyone. Therefore, it's important to work with someone who understands your biochemistry and can fill in the blanks, so to speak, in *your* deficiencies.

What to Eat? Let's Make This Simple

There is no lack of evidence to support the notion that our food choices affect our health. And most of my clients notice that once they feel better physically, they think more clearly and feel more *emotionally* sound!

Most people instinctively know what to eat. The guidelines have been paved by common sense and experts for centuries:

1. Eat your vegetables.
2. Eat your fruits.
3. Eat your fiber.
4. Avoid sugar and foods devoid of nutrients.
5. Eat healthy fats and proteins.
6. Eat real food. This means that you should consume food found in nature, not processed or packaged synthetic "food" full of chemical preservatives. Whole, real foods will nourish your body because the body can work with them and assimilate their potent, healthful constituents.
7. Drink clean water.

8. If you feel ill or just "bad" after eating a particular a food, you may want to avoid it. On the other hand, if there's a food that makes you feel great after eating it, continue to include it in your diet.
9. Most people do better without gluten, soy, and processed chemicals in their food.

And above all, remember that diet is more than just finding the perfect balanced ratios and following them militantly. It's about listening to your body and allowing it to guide you by its symptoms – seeing what works and what doesn't work. If you need help in distinguishing this, that's what naturopathic and functional doctors are here for.

CHAPTER 4

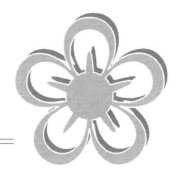

Moving Toward Healthier Outcomes

With the current obesity epidemic, it's no surprise that one of the biggest goals men and women set for themselves at *any* time of the year is weight loss. Unfortunately, it's also no surprise that the methods by which many go about obtaining this goal has a lousy track record of maintained success. This is for various reasons, including those mentioned in the last chapter, ranging from cravings to confusion from information overload!

When biochemical cravings trump rational thinking, many forego moderate lifestyle adjustments and desperately reach for a quick fix. Over the years, many of my clients have come to me after various dieting attempts. They express frustration with the extreme methods required to follow such militant food plans. They miserably report failed attempts to maintain weight loss from fad starvation diets, hamster-wheel workouts, and ingesting pills that shut down their internal hunger cues.

Initially, these approaches can and will create change, but usually only for short periods of time. Why do these methods continually fail in helping people to achieve optimal body weight? Two big reasons:

1. Most of them focus only on making an individual *look* better, not *feel* better.
2. They rely on extreme methods that cannot be kept up for the long haul.

Any big change, especially in health, requires integration of the whole person. Unless we are ready to deal with how we will be affected emotionally by releasing our self-destructive habits, the angst from perceiving a life without these numbing habits can prevent one from moving forward. Brad Lamm, author of *Just Ten Pounds, Easy Steps to Weighing what you Want (Finally)*,[1] has a simple and elegant way of expressing this fact: "Change is uncomfortable."

Our society is one in which entertainment and busy-ness are used to distract ourselves from feeling anything but elation. We often prefer numbness to any type of "negative" feeling. Where weight loss is concerned, the desired change is usually so extreme that most people can't fathom how to release their various self-made prisons and dietary rules all by themselves. They need some support and a rational, objective guide.

For example, emotions that were suppressed with excessive food consumption can become uncovered while shedding pounds. An understanding and loving support system can serve as a foundation as one literally releases old weight and habits and forms a new identity. I've found clinically that any attempt at extreme weight loss will ultimately fail if this emotional support is not in place, especially for women.

I consider it important to honor what brings my clients joy as we work to alleviate suffering from years of perceived failures. Where weight loss is concerned, this does not entail a "diet police" mentality or any other tough love method. These methods tend to have the same effect on us as listening to a motivational speaker jump around on stage shouting encouraging words, and then, at the end of the day, returning to our "real" lives, feeling empty and unmotivated.

Weight Loss the Integrative Way

Once proper emotional support is in place, the next step in achieving change is follow-through. This starts by reestablishing proper signaling from the brain to the hand that holds the fork or reaches for the refrigerator door! What is not recognized in conventional weight loss plans is the importance of modulating this intricate biochemical signaling process.

According to Dr. Amen, low activity in the brain's cingulate gyrus could account for why some of us get stuck in self-defeating behavior. This portion of the brain is responsible for "shifting gears," and it needs to be engaged in order to change.

One treatment option is to supply the body with precursors and nutrients needed for proper brain signaling. As a naturopathic doctor, I believe that it's also important to address why specific brain-signaling molecules might be deficient to begin with.

In weight loss resistance, certain hunger cues can also become imbalanced. Unless this is regulated, your willpower will be in a boxing match with your biochemistry. The fight will be between your vow to avoid temptations and an inability to stop your hand from reaching for that yummy "treat," and we know how that fight ends!

A study in the *Journal of Clinical Investigation* looked at this pattern and suggested that leptin resistance may be a key player in this rematch:

> *Specifically, hypothalamic activity and activity in areas of the brain involved in emotional (cingulate gyrus; Brodmann area [BA]) and cognitive (middle frontal gyrus) control are commonly engaged in states of*

> *leptin sufficiency and leptin repletion ... The pivotal role for leptin in the CNS-mediated responses to the maintenance of reduced weight is also demonstrated by the neural activity observed during the state of relative hypoleptinemia following weight loss relative to subjects at usual weight and leptin levels ... The regions include insula, cingulate gyrus, medial frontal gyrus, precuneus, middle occipital gyrus, superior frontal gyrus, and superior temporal gyrus.*[2]

The researchers in this study demonstrated that dieters who accomplish weight loss may have a biological backlash, and overeat due to a "relative leptin deficiency." By injecting the struggling dieters with this appetite-suppressing hormone, emotional control, decision making, and the brain's executive function were restored, thereby improving their signaling cues for hunger and their control over eating.

This means that your blood sugar, digestion, and brain all have to work together. But wait, there's more! ...

One last piece of weight loss-related biochemistry was explored in the *Yale Journal of Biological Medicine*.[3] It appears that carrying excess weight can be due to a faulty food-pleasure feedback mechanism in the brain.

In this particular study,[3] researchers assessed how foods affected the reward center in the brains of overweight volunteers versus control subjects. It was found that following the ingestion of a sugary treat, obese individuals tend to have less activation in the reward portion of their brain. This finding adds to the above discussion on leptin and offers another possible explanation for compulsive eating, as it seems the brain responds differently to satiety and satisfaction cues in those who carry excess pounds.

Another important part of this discussion is the significance of "the real thing." In terms of sweeteners, it appears that you can't fool the brain. Studies suggest that artificial sweeteners do not alleviate cravings and can actually *increase* rebound weight gain and food urges.[4]

Our biochemistry is clearly affected by what we eat. Our brains, in return, influence our future food choices. Addressing all of these interacting biochemical pathways can mean the difference between knowing what to do and actually doing it! In fact, to me this is THE important component in the laundry list of "avoid" and "include" grocery list items. When the head, heart, and hand are at peace with each other, one can expect to leave the grocery store smiling instead of scowling!

What About Genes (not Jeans)?

Good news for those who feel that their weight is their genetic destiny. It's not your genes that dictate your health and weight, but rather the *expression* of your genes. You have the ability to easily turn genes on and off with your lifestyle and emotional state. One simple way to do this is through movement. According to Dr. Mercola,[5]

> *One such example has to do with genetic markers that may make you more prone to obesity. You can very effectively reduce the effects of these genes by increasing your physical activity.*
>
> *According to researchers from Great Britain's Medical Research Council in Cambridge, regular exercise reduces the genetic tendency toward obesity by 40 percent!*
>
> *A separate study among Amish people also found those who had the FTO gene [the gene that carries the potential for obesity] but were very physically active weighed about the same as others who did not carry the gene.*[5]

You may have noticed this with friends who have both obese and non-obese family members. Chances are that the heavy members of the family were not engaged in a healthy lifestyle. Still, don't let an obsession with exercise become a replacement for food fundamentalism, or think that by moving your booty, you can now get away with harming your body with non-nurturing foods. We'll address this topic next.

Lead Your Own Weigh!

The media is adept at glorifying famous celebrities and portraying hand-picked medical "authorities" as health experts to the public. Unfortunately, not all of these "gurus" have achieved book sales based on wellness education, integrative health skills, or clinical excellence. The result is popular dietary trends from various marketing ploys that lead many astray down a crazed weight loss path. It's a modern-day "Alice down the rabbit hole." One can get vertigo watching the ping-pong match between vegan diet worshipers and Paleolithic diet devotees, each group touting its side with religious fervor.

Nowadays, it's not enough to question everything that goes into our mouths; we also have to validate which exercise party to campaign for. We purchase pedometers and software to form charts, plot our progress, and calculate the exact rate of our warm-up, peak, and cool-down. (Thank God our electronic devices now have a calculator, stopwatch, and heart rate monitor all-in-one, or we'd fall over from the weight of all of our gadgets!) I picture us in the future, walking through the gym door in something resembling a space suit that magically absorbs sweat and stench and increases calories burned by 200 percent on the treadmill, such that we only have to walk for two minutes to obtain optimal results.

With our manic society approaching an obesity epidemic, we haven't paused long enough to consider that reaching frantically for another "diet" book may not be the best solution to our life-long lifestyle problem. Unfortunately, we get lost in a societal programming to finish this rat race competition to achieve the ultimate outward appearance.

If there really was a panacea diet for weight loss, a perfect form of exercise for a celebrity body, and a super pill for the fountain of youth, then why isn't everyone thin and youthful?

The question of how we can keep up our frantic lifestyle as we follow the latest new trend, yet also have a perfect figure with the least amount of effort, is becoming what exercise is all about. Surprise, surprise, it's not working!

According to the CDC:

> *American society has become 'obesogenic,' characterized by environments that promote increased food intake, nonhealthful foods, and physical inactivity.*[6]

A 2010 report in JAMA stated that approximately one-third of adults are overweight.[7] This translates to 30 percent of the adult population having a body mass index (BMI) equal to or greater than 30. Since 1980, obesity rates have doubled in adults and tripled in children.

The National Heart, Lung, and Blood Institute reports:

> *As a major contributor to preventive death in the United States today, overweight and obesity pose a major public health challenge.*[8]

So, now it's not enough for chronic dieters to feel crummy about their failure from following the trends and formulas to a tee. Now their guilt is also increasing as they feel blamed for consuming the addictive foods and dietary trends that are promoted in the first place. Yikes!

The Best (Blood) Type of Workout?

So, what's the answer for the best workout regimen? Dr. Peter D'Adamo, a naturopathic doctor and author of several bestselling blood type diet books, believes that blood type and temperament are the keys to successful outcomes in the areas of diet and exercise.[9] As an integrative practitioner, naturopathic doctor, and functional medicine practitioner, you know my line by now. I, too, believe that the "ideal workout" is based on the individual. Just as the same diet won't work for everyone, the same exercise won't either.

> Here are some Blood Type specific workout tips from Des Depass, a personal fitness trainer who uses this concept when working with others. He provides an example of how different exercises for different blood types (associated with different temperaments) may be more ideal than a one-size-fits-all approach.[10]
>
> **Blood Type O** individuals should incorporate resistance training, including heavy lifting and short burst exercises that require extreme energy. Lighter lifting with 15-minute bursts as hard as possible are recommended for cardiovascular workouts, followed by a short break.
>
> **Type O sample workout:**
> Circuit training that combines calisthenics and weight lifting constitutes an effective cardiovascular workout. An example of a circuit would be squats with or without a dumbbell or barbell added for more difficulty, also add pushups and bicep curls with a two-minute break in between. It is recommended to string together as many exercises as possible using light-to-medium weights. By keeping the heart rate up, body fat loss will be noticeable right away. Des Depass recommends that Type O's should stick with eating the

foods recommended for their blood type post-workout, and to stay hydrated in order to prevent crashing. (References for foods that are beneficial for different blood types and conditions can be found in Dr. D'Adamo's, "Eat Right 4 Your Type" publications. For example, Type O's thrive on meats, poultry, and healthy fats such as olive oil.)

Blood Type A individuals need exercises for stress modulation. Examples include kettle bells, boxing, martial arts, or other stress-busting workouts. Gardening and carpentry can be a beneficial combo of cardio and strength training. Light running, core work, and bodyweight movement can be used for light days.

Type A sample workout:
Boxing, focused breathing exercises such as yoga or tai chi, and kettle bells are very beneficial. These help Type A individuals focus and relieve stress while burning calories. It is recommended to make sure proper technique is used to avoid injury. Alternatives are housework, construction, or intensive gardening, if exercise is too exhausting for stressed-out Type A folks.

Blood Type B exercises are based on genotype, which is a newer addition to Dr. D'Adamo's blood-type diet work. This classifies individuals into six different genotypes (Hunters, Gatherers, Nomads, Teachers, Explorers, and Warriors) by combining blood type with genetic survival strategies that correspond to external traits, such as body type, jaw shape, and teeth patterns. Exercise for Type Bs will be different based on their genotypes.

Type B sample workout:
One genotype of blood type B, known as a Gatherer, is recommended to use mostly balance work for focus and centering. Examples of exercises to incorporate include long bike rides, 45 minutes of

elliptical machines on random settings, weight lifting with dumbbell exercises consisting of standing triceps extensions, bicep curls, shoulder presses, or Bosu Ball workouts.

Blood Type AB is the rarest blood type and not as well studied by this fitness expert. However, it seems that almost any type of exercise but heavy lifting works well for this blood type.

Type AB sample workout:
This could consist of combining the focus exercises of blood Type A with the balancing benefits of Type B workouts. For example:
Day 1: Yoga
Day 2: Bike ride
Day 3: Yoga
Day 4: Bike ride
Day 5: Tai chi and light boxing
Day 6: Bike ride
Day 7: Light dumbbell work at a slow, controlled pace.
The goal is balance, moderation, and moderate intensity for blood type AB. They should incorporate focused breathing techniques to center and prepare the body for the workout, and finish with stretching and breathing to calm the body and relax the mind.

I wanted to give my brilliant predecessor such a highlighted focus on individualized exercise for a variety of reasons:

1. Dr. D'Adamo is a genius. I believe that he has been overlooked by many people simply due to the letters "ND" (as opposed to "MD") following his name.
2. Dr. D'Adamo is a naturopathic physician who practices generative medicine. Instead of pursuing a career based on peer prestige by staying within the confines of conventionally accepted research, Dr. D'Adamo has pursued a line of work that stretches scientific reasoning beyond the bottom line.

He provides insight into a different paradigm that considers biochemical variations and focuses on clinical outcomes.

3. Within my own understanding of functional medicine, I incorporate blood type and genotype into my practice and get positive clinical results. I further individualize this approach to include factors such as ethnicity, genetic predisposition, disease history, nutrigenomics, enjoyment, and individual capabilities. I also find the framework of Ayurvedic doshas – the three types of bodily constitutions explained in this ancient form of medicine – helpful in recommending different types of yoga practices for different clients.

Debunking the All-Inclusive Use of the Latest Trend

The latest trend for fat-burning is peak exercise, also known as interval training. A good amount of current research seems to be aimed at supporting its use for all. I admit, the results of these trials are impressive, and I use the technique myself. (It fits my blood type profile).

Still, as noted above, individualized exercise should ultimately be based on what will best suit the participant, not solely on generalized studies. For example, in those who have chronic fatigue and burnout, peak exercise could be counterproductive. This excessive movement can result in increased mobilization of inflammatory mediators that a tired body simply can't eliminate; this can also happen in those who have sufficient energy metabolism.

In this scenario, the effect could actually result in weight gain, as more fat is produced to sequester mobilized toxicants that could create damage elsewhere in the body. This is because your body cares more about your survival than the ten extra pounds that make you crazy.

Therefore, for these fatigued clients who burn the candle at both ends, regardless of what the studies say, biochemistry and their individualized needs support the use of *gentle* exercise. The effectiveness of this approach in inflamed individuals was studied by York University.

In this study, yoga was found to be beneficial not only for weight loss, but for arthritic pains and mental/emotional health symptoms in those with fibromyalgia. The investigators, according to *Science Daily*,[11] reported that this form of yoga actually increases cortisol, which is anti-inflammatory and dysregulated in those who suffer from this disease:

> A new study by York University researchers finds that practicing yoga reduces the physical and psychological symptoms of chronic pain in women with fibromyalgia. The study is the first to look at the effects of yoga on cortisol levels in women with fibromyalgia. The condition, which predominantly affects women, is characterized by chronic pain and fatigue; common symptoms include muscle stiffness, sleep disturbances, gastrointestinal discomfort, anxiety and depression.[11]

According to an article from the *Chopra Newsletter*, there are additional emotional and cognitive benefits of yoga.[12] The article states that the greatest benefits of yoga can be found by relaxing into a pose, not forcing oneself into a stretch. This is accomplished by pausing once an individual's point of resistance is found, and then breathing into it rather than using force to move beyond it. This gentle approach teaches patience, awareness of the body's feedback, and to acknowledge and work through limitations that block a person from his or her goals.

It is believed that the more we embrace and surrender to our limits through the practice of yoga, the more effectively we can evaluate them and strategize how to overcome them. This practice of union leads one away from reactionary responses to stressors, and instead into peaceful and calm resolutions. This is "food" for the hyperactive nervous system and allows for healing of the whole body. By calming stress feedback to the brain, hormones are better balanced and the ability of yoga to promote weight loss and boost energy is easier to understand.

And finally, a Finnish study[13] provided evidence for the often-overlooked yet powerful effect of outdoor physical activity on stress reduction and weight loss:

> *Restorative experiences in favorite exercise and activity outdoor areas, waterside environments and extensively managed natural settings (mainly urban woodlands) were stronger than in favorite places in built urban settings or green spaces in urban settings (mostly parks) ... The more worries about money and work...a person had, the more stressed a person had felt during the last year, the less energetic s/he had felt, the lower was the number of visits to the favorite place...and the lower the typical level of restorative experiences.*[13]

It seems that the more you are feeling stressed, depressed, or frazzled, the harder but even more important it is to get yourself into the woods ... or at least into a calm and natural state.

Don't Forget ... Love Yourself

My final suggestion on this subject: If what you are doing isn't working for you, try something different, not more of the same. Consider tuning into your body, enjoying your movement, and going inside yourself for the answer to these questions: Is it your serotonin-deficient brain making a nonsensical suggestion to not move when your body would actually benefit from the endorphin rush? Or, is your body burned out, inflamed, and being "big ol' cranky pants"? If you listen, your body will guide you. If you're not that in-tune yet, try alternating physical activities with relaxation, and compare how you feel after each.

Also, be flexible. Your ideal form of exercise could change with time. I'm finding that, for both myself and my clients, when the focus changes from seeking external perfection to health and self-care, amazing results follow.

Finally, no matter what form you choose, there is good scientific evidence of benefits from any type of movement, especially for reducing the health risks associated with too much sitting. A study in the *International Journal of Epidemiology* reported that even moderate activity lowers all-cause mortality.[14] Other benefits of exercise include better brain function, reduced inflammation, and stress relief.

Not everyone is meant to be a size 2, but we all have a natural state of wellness in which we feel good and our bodies hum contentedly. As discussed, there are many factors that, when balanced, create optimal weight results that far surpass ultimate failures from dietary restriction, deprivation, and excessive exercise. In my practice, addressing the reasons why one feels the need to lose weight is a key factor in maintaining lasting results. In this way, one can shift beliefs from a fear-based, rat-race mentality toward productive thoughts and actions that are consistent with a health-oriented lifestyle.

Remember, you don't have to struggle alone. Consider consulting an expert ... a doctor who will listen to you and your needs, who knows your history, temperament, biochemistry, and your specific current health concerns. I suggest a practitioner who has training in functional medicine, knowledge in balancing neurotransmitters, experience in integrating genetic bio-individuality, and who uses an approach that embraces organ system biology. These biochemistry whizzes can help decipher exactly what to do to biologically set you up for success and end your battle of the bulge.

In the end, making desperate attempts to achieve the perfect body, which are sought outside of one's own inner wisdom, or chasing panaceas based on marketing ploys, will only produce short-term changes in one's ultimate goal of peace and lasting change in one's health. My hope in writing this book is that you can bless yourself with the gift of honoring your biochemical uniqueness throughout this journey toward a healthier, happier, harmonious life.

In the upcoming chapters, I will be focusing on an organ system approach of bringing balance to the body. I will be discussing specific tools that can be implemented along the way to achieve optimal health outcomes. Still, keep in mind that bio-individuality should be the ultimate determinant in creating your health plan, beyond any generalized "expert" advice.

If these or any other suggestions don't feel right in your gut (literally and figuratively), honor that, stop, and discuss it with that well-respected integrative physician who is supporting your growth. It could be that your body needs support to process certain suggestions, to slow down and catch up with healing, or that your body might do better with another suggestion altogether.

Figuratively speaking, many people say that the gut has wisdom, and they are right. In the next chapter, you'll discover just how vital it is to have a happy digestive tract in order to run everything else more smoothly.

CHAPTER 5

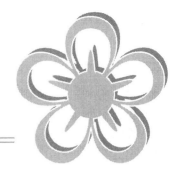

Your Gut: The Home of Mood, Food, and Immunity

It may seem like an obvious statement that everything in the body is connected. Yet, in a medical paradigm that has focused on specialists and the isolation of body parts, this is not the norm. In fact, the origin of your symptoms might not stem from the dysfunctional organ at all! That organ might actually be an innocent bystander forced into action after being affected by a distant mechanism gone awry in your body. Still, it's hard to find a conventional doctor who will look beyond his or her area of body part expertise and view the individual as operating within a wider system. This is not because these doctors aren't intelligent, it's because of how they are trained to think.

In naturopathic medical school, we are taught to honor the body's symptoms as its unique means of communication. When the body speaks its wisdom through sensations, we are either pleased with the feeling or we're anxious to make it stop! When pain or discomfort predominates, the body is signaling that something needs attention.

That's where your functional medicine and naturopathic practitioners come in. We can serve as your translators of this seemingly foreign language.

In fact, most diagnoses are symptoms of an underlying SYSTEMIC (whole-body) malfunction. Therefore, suppressing an organ that is speaking out is counter to the principle, "treat the cause." There's an ancient adage in naturopathic medicine that is drilled into our heads as young and bright-eyed medical students. "When in doubt, treat the gut." The reason for this valuable advice is that your digestive tract is a key player in most of your body's communication processes, including pain signaling, immune function, hormonal balance, nutrient assimilation, mood support, and much more!

Ever hear the expression, "If mamma ain't happy, no one is"? Well, if your gut is angry, your whole body can run amuck, and this can happen even without getting digestive symptoms. Your gut's "anger" could come out sideways as imbalances in hormones, inflammation, or undesirable weight.

It's estimated that 60-80 percent of the immune system and over 70 percent of our neurotransmitters (chemical signaling molecules responsible for all sorts of reactions in the nervous system) reside in the gastrointestinal tract. As mentioned earlier, the gut has a specific name for its own nervous system (the *enteric nervous system,* or *ENS*), and also for its immune system (the *gut-associated lymphoid tissue*, or *GALT*). The ENS interacts with many different enzymes and hormones to send feedback to your brain. Meanwhile, the GALT helps manage your immune system's reactions.

Since the gastrointestinal tract is such a powerful and large organ, you might think it would be protected from damage. Unfortunately, this is not true. The gut barrier is just *one cell thick* and can be damaged by numerous factors common to everyday living. Furthermore, with the advent of "better living through chemistry," our digestive tracts are under constant daily attack from new foreign species. These include:

- medications such as nonsteroidal anti-inflammatory drugs (NSAIDs), antibiotics, and cytotoxic agents (chemotherapy)
- food sensitivities or allergies resulting from processed and chemicalized foods
- excessive alcohol or addictive substances
- trauma
- decreased digestive enzyme output due to chronic external or internal stressors
- chronic psychological stress
- underlying inflammation from various factors, including disease processes, blood sugar imbalances, bacteria, viruses, or parasites

The gut is the major interface of communication, in charge of determining what is or isn't harmful to the body. Thus, when the gut is damaged, the immune system becomes dysregulated, feedback to the brain gets distorted, and absorption and assimilation of nutrients diminish. This results in lower production of health promoting building blocks at the cellular level and causes many systemic issues, which we'll discuss later in this chapter.

Leaky Gut

Malabsorption and increased intestinal permeability (a.k.a. "leaky gut") are two issues that can result from sustained damage to the gastrointestinal lining. This damage causes breakdown of the intestinal lining and decreases its ability to filter out and protect the body from unwanted bacteria and toxins. Without proper filtering, these little critters and byproducts can squeeze through gaps between the intestinal cells and be re-released into the bloodstream. This can result in a wide array of uncomfortable symptoms, allergies, and autoimmune conditions.

Along with reduced filtering ability, damage to intestinal cells can also reduce the surface area required for absorption of nutrients and other helpful biological substances. This decrease in nutrient availability can cause a host of other symptoms, including changes in appetite.

The gut communicates its hunger signals through hormones, e.g., insulin and leptin, to the hypothalamus, which is the portion of the brain that regulates survival instincts such as hunger. Without proper absorption, nutrients that make these signals possible are missing. The result is a breakdown in this gut-brain communication, leading to intense food cravings and overeating because of an inability to feel satiated, or full.

If intestinal tract disorders are preventing the body from absorbing complex foods, it will naturally yearn for what I label "extreme foods," like sugar, caffeine, and processed foods. The body craves these substances because it is unable to absorb more complex and nutrient-dense foods. However, junk foods can't sustain a healthy body. Although they appear to be sources of quick energy, they can promote eventual cellular fatigue from extremes in blood sugar, and can create a cycle of dependence. Furthermore, extreme foods can actually intensify nutrient deficiencies and resulting cravings.

For example, processed sugar is devoid of any mineral, vitamin, or other form of sustenance. It can also rob the body of essential components due to being processed more like a drug than a food. If an individual is already healthy with a strong digestive tract and a balanced nutrient intake, an occasional sugary treat can be digested and enjoyed with no problem. However, for the unfortunate person with a permeable gut lining, this same treat can trigger any of the symptoms discussed above.

Processed foods can also be harmful by causing digestive insult. They are not only devoid of nutrients, but also contain many chemicals that can further damage the intestinal lining, thus perpetuating this vicious cycle of cravings and further nutrient depletion.

Because of the gut's multiple roles in health, malabsorption also causes a host of other symptoms, including:

- stomach or intestinal pain/discomfort, gas, bloating
- low mood, decreased energy, or cloudy thinking
- joint pain
- hormonal imbalances
- low tolerance for stress
- skin rashes

The first step in healing your gut lining is to replace fast foods with nutritious, whole, healthy foods that can assist in healing. If you are addicted to a processed food, then supporting your biochemistry and emotional health, as discussed in the previous chapter, can help.

Fortunately, it's possible to pinpoint various contributors to the perpetuation of leaky gut issues once the diet is cleaned up. I also usually recommend specific lab tests to rule out any major issues and to help verify improvement in biochemical markers along with symptom relief.

Intestinal permeability can be evaluated through various tests such as a comprehensive digestive stool analysis and specialized functional laboratory assessments. In addition, through the assessment of other markers, an integrative practitioner can evaluate a person for food sensitivities, inflammatory processes in the gut, intestinal overgrowth or other intestinal dysfunction, nutrient deficiencies, and hormonal and neurological imbalances. These tests, along with a case history, provide a good basis for how to proceed in addressing weight concerns, cravings, and any other chronic symptoms.

Different People, Different Causes

As noted above, leaky gut is caused by a variety of factors and can result in multiple symptoms. Therefore, a one-size-fits-all approach will not work. For example, let's take a look at the embarrassing situation of excess gas and bloating.

In one scenario, you might notice that you become flatulent and bloated only after eating. In this case, you might lack the enzymes needed to break down certain substances in your diet. As the undigested food is fermented by bacteria in your large bowel, gas accumulates. One way to address this is to use a high-quality digestive enzyme with meals. For those who are willing to dig more deeply for the root cause and to implement preventative medicine, the appropriate lifestyle and nutritional support that addresses the cause of the low enzyme availability (such as stress, nutrient depletion, and medication side effects) can also be implemented.

On the other hand, for another "windy" individual, the issue could be an undiagnosed food sensitivity, allergy, or bacterial overgrowth that causes irritation to the gastrointestinal tract. In this case, the use of demulcent herbal therapies to soothe and coat the digestive tract, anti-inflammatory nutrients, anti-microbials, and individualized nutritional support to correct resultant deficiencies would be the best approach.

System-Wide Breakdowns

As discussed, when the body can't effectively break down a substance (whether due to a lack of digestive enzymes or to food sensitivities/allergies), an inflammatory response can ensue. These undigested proteins are viewed by the body as "foreign," hence are attacked by the immune system. An internal inflammatory response will ignite the gut, thereby compromising its barrier. As a result, the incompletely digested proteins can leak through the permeable gut membrane and escape, triggering a systemic, chronic and low-grade inflammatory response. Over time, this will cause long-term energy and nutrient deficits. This can lead to chronic illness, including autoimmune disorders.

In autoimmunity, when the body's immune cells respond by attacking these "food invaders" (which are usually complexes of undigested peptides), they can get "confused" and attack your own tissues as well! In other words, compromised digestion sets the stage for immune over-reactivity and what might appear to the sufferer as unrelated symptoms.

Many people still believe that the lack of noticeable digestive reactions to a food must mean that their bodies agree with it. Research, however, suggests that this isn't necessarily the case.

In 2002, an article[1] from the *Journal of Neurology, Neurosurgery, & Psychiatry* reported the following link between dietary proteins and non-digestive-related complaints:

> *It has taken nearly 2000 years to appreciate that a common dietary protein introduced to the human diet relatively late in evolutionary terms (some 10 000 years ago), can produce human disease not only of the gut but also the skin and the nervous system. The protean neurological manifestations of gluten sensitivity can occur without gut involvement and neurologists must therefore become familiar with the common neurological presentations and means of diagnosis of this disease.*[1]

Sayer Ji's article, "Opening Pandora's Box: The Clinical Role of Wheat in Human Disease,"[2] is a wonderful read that links the concept of food lectins (made popular by the Blood Type Diet) with nutrigenomics. (See Chapter 4 for more information on nutrigenomics). Sayer Ji illustrates this concept using the wheat lectin.

Wheat is very hard to digest, due to its protective outer coating. Moreover, the lectin in wheat (WGA) can cause damage to various tissues in the body, initiating inflammation and leading to diseases that extend beyond the gastrointestinal tract.

Sayer Ji feels that this WGA lectin may be the reason why populations that consume a large amount of wheat have seen a significant rise in chronic inflammatory and degenerative conditions.[2] This is true even when allergies or intolerances are not obvious. Below he explains how this compound can act as an immune provoker and how this may scientifically explain why wheat can wreak such havoc on a variety of organ systems:

> *The time has come to draw attention to the powerful little chemical in wheat known as 'wheat germ agglutinin' (WGA) which is largely responsible for many of wheat's pervasive, and difficult to diagnose, ill effects. Not only does WGA throw a monkey wrench into our assumptions about the primary causes of wheat intolerance, it also pulls the rug out from under one of the health food industry's favorite poster children since high concentrations of WGA [are] found in "whole wheat," including its supposedly superior sprouted form.*
>
> *What is unique about WGA is that it can do direct damage to the majority of tissues in the human body without requiring a specific set of genetic susceptibilities and/or immune-mediated articulations.*[2]

The WGA glycoprotein component of wheat is only one reason why so many people experience variable problems from wheat consumption. In fact, it is the gliadin peptide molecule that is usually studied and correlated to various health issues in regards to this popular grain. According to the American Academy of Allergy, Asthma & Immunology,

> Antigliadin and antiendomysial (transglutaminase) antibodies have been studied extensively in gluten-sensitive enteropathy. The presence of antigliadin antibodies strongly suggests that gluten-sensitive enteropathy is due, in part, to a dietary element. Both serum and secretory levels of IgA are increased, whereas IgG levels are only minimally elevated and the IgM level is often decreased.[3]

According to the NY Academy of Sciences, wheat enteropathy (damage to the intestinal lining from an immune response to wheat) can be linked to some cases of multiple sclerosis:[4]

> We determined the level of serum immunoglobulin A and immunoglobulin G antigliadin and antitissue transglutaminase [anti-tTG] antibodies in 98 patients with multiple sclerosis. We found a highly significant increase in titers of immunoglobulin G antibodies against gliadin and tissue transglutaminase in the multiple sclerosis patients. Seven patients had a positive IgG AGA [antigliadin antibodies], whereas only 2 controls presented positive titers (P = 0.03). Four patients had positive IgG anti-tTG while all the controls tested negative (P = 0.02).

Many other studies link various other symptoms and chronic diseases, such as rheumatoid arthritis and other autoimmune disorders, to leaky gut caused by chronic irritation to the gastrointestinal mucosa. A review paper in *The New England Journal of Medicine* lists 55 "diseases" that can result from eating gluten.[5] These include osteoporosis, irritable bowel disease, anemia, cancer, fatigue, canker sores, rheumatoid arthritis, lupus, multiple sclerosis, inflammatory bowel disease, and almost all other autoimmune diseases.

Furthermore, a 2005 article published in *BMC Psychiatry* discusses how the gluten protein in wheat, rye, and barley can negatively affect hormonal balance and neurotransmitters in the brain.[6] It follows that food sensitivities can affect brain health as well. Gluten has also been linked to many psychiatric and neurological diseases, including anxiety, depression, dementia, migraines, epilepsy, and neuropathy (nerve damage). It has also been linked to autism.

Many may wonder, "If gluten has so many negative effects, why do those who have problems from it still eat it?" The answer is they may not be able to easily stop! WGA has opioid-like properties, which make it not only non-nutritive (for most of us who are sensitive), but also addictive.[2]

> *These pharmacologically active, opiate-like proteins in gluten are known as gluten exorphins (A5, B4, B5, C) and gliadorphins. In the short term, they may anesthetize us to the long term, adverse effects of WGA. Gluten also contains exceptionally high levels of the excitotoxic l-aspartic and l-glutamic amino acids, which can also be highly addictive, not unlike their synthetic shadow molecules aspartame and monosodium glutamate.*[2]

Food sensitivities can also increase cravings through their effects on blood sugar. Eating problematic foods triggers an immune response and ignites inflammation in the gut. This creates fluctuating levels of glucose in the body as the body attempts to stabilize itself. The resulting spikes and dips in cellular glucose availability creates an addictive cycle as one tries to regulate them by consuming more of the offending food. I've heard this cycle referred to as the "feed me or I'll kill you" syndrome.

Recently, a well-known doctor, Alessio Fasano, broke new bounds in research when he demonstrated how gluten affects the protein in the body that regulates intestinal permeability in everyone, not just in those who are sensitive.[7] If enough stressors hit any individual, increased permeability can eventually result. For this reason, many practitioners recommend that everyone avoid this sticky food substance.

Celiac Disease versus Gluten Sensitivity

I talked in Chapter 3 about the different possible ways that our bodies can react to gluten – as an autoimmune reaction (which includes celiac and non-intestinal gluten reactions in genetically-susceptible individuals); as an allergic reaction (usually a wheat allergy), or as a reaction that doesn't involve the immune system at all. Although some of the same terms are sometimes used to describe different types of gluten reactions (which makes things confusing!), we'll call this last kind of reaction "gluten sensitivity" for the sake of simplicity.[8]

Researchers have hypothesized that in people with autoimmune gluten reactions, their genetic susceptibility can influence levels of immune mediators, receptor function, and even permeability of the intestine. Specific gene sequences, such as HLA-DQ2 and HLA-DQ8, are often tested when a patient is suspected of having gluten-related problems. The presence of one or both of these markers confirms genetic predisposition to *autoimmune* gluten reactions, and highly correlates with celiac disease.

However, environment also plays a role in gluten reactions. Environmental factors include nutrient deficiencies and certain medications, such as NSAIDs (non-steroidal anti-inflammatory drugs), which increase intestinal permeability in many individuals. One expert suggests:

> *This may explain why in up to 5% of all cases of classically defined celiac disease the typical HLA-DQ haplotypes*

> [combinations of HLA-DQ genotypes] are not found. However, determining the factors associated [with] greater or lesser degrees of susceptibility to gliadin's intrinsically toxic effect should be...secondary to the fact that it is has been demonstrated to be toxic to both non-celiacs and celiacs.[9]

A recent large study[10] looked at almost 30,000 patients from 1969 to 2008 and examined deaths in three groups: subjects with full-blown celiac disease (including intestinal atrophy), subjects with intestinal inflammation but no intestinal atrophy, and subjects with "latent" celiac disease (elevated gluten and/or celiac antibodies, but a normal intestinal lining). The findings were surprising. Those with celiac disease had a 39 percent increased risk of death. A 35 percent increased risk was found in those who only showed an immune response to gluten, and a 72 percent increased risk was found in those with gut inflammation associated gluten exposure!

These findings suggest that you don't have to have full-blown celiac disease (as confirmed by a positive intestinal biopsy) to experience various, and sometimes serious health problems from eating gluten. Yet, a large number of individuals who develop problems from eating gluten don't even know it, assuming instead that other factors are responsible for their symptoms. Problems from gluten can be completely prevented when one is made aware of the danger.

Although it is true that there is no definitive lab test for food sensitivities, in general, since they differ from true allergies, there are clues that a skilled practitioner can hone in on. True food allergies are an immediate response mediated by the immunoglobulin IgE, whereas food sensitivities are typically delayed reactions that involve a different set of immunoglobulins: IgG, IgM, and/or IgA. In my clinic, I recommend a celiac profile for every client, as even slightly elevated serum antibody levels can provide clues of a sensitivity reaction. Finding a practitioner that can help support you with either type of reaction is important.

Integrative practitioners are now also using non-conventional tests for identifying food sensitivities including ALCAT testing or IgG patterns. There are also tests available that measure cross-reactivity reactions between gluten antibodies and certain foods other than gluten. However, any of these lab tests should be used in combination with the "gold standard" – the elimination diet challenge. This involves the elimination of all possible food allergens for three to four weeks. After this time period, one would introduce a category of food, one at time, into the diet. For example, Day 1 might be gluten day. Following the challenge of introducing this one food, watch for any negative effects on mood, sleep, or digestive disturbances for three days.

Remember that the gut affects the whole system; therefore, also note any other vague symptoms, such as fatigue, brain fog, aches and pains, insomnia, and heart palpitations, any of which could result from gluten ingestion. After the initial three days, if there is still uncertainty as to whether gluten is the cause of a physical discomfort, have a "gluten-feast-all-out-day" and observe again for the next three days. Any negative response will be heightened and can help confirm that the body is negatively impacted by gluten. The three-day time span is needed for the immune system to respond to an offending food. (This also illustrates why eating a variety of foods can prevent the immune system from becoming sensitive to one substance).

If there are other suspected food sensitivities, ensuring that any aggravation from gluten is completely resolved before introducing the next category is important. Then follow the same process outlined above. It is best to use pure forms of the food so as not to confuse which food is causing a reaction. For example, to test gluten it would be best to eat pure wheat cereal than to consume a gluten-dairy-sugar-filled baked good containing wheat. Using this method of elimination and reintroduction will help to determine whether symptoms are related to diet, and can empower one to make different choices if needed.

Moderation is Key

Does all this talk about the inflammatory potential of wheat mean that we are doomed to never eat out again or never again partake in Mom's homemade wheat pasta? It depends on the person.

I feel that, if the body is healthy, moderation is the answer. If you already know that you have celiac disease, or have symptoms plus the genetic predisposition for celiac, it's important that you *strictly* avoid gluten, and on a permanent basis. An individualized approach makes it possible to catch a gluten sensitivity early and prevent significant health problems – including celiac disease – down the road.

I have found that once most people go the route of saying no to gluten, they tend to *stay* gluten-free because they feel better and have more energy. Some even report that they no longer like the taste of gluten-filled foods after taking a vacation from it. I love hearing this. I have heard some experts proclaim that if you can stop a food for three weeks, you can literally transform your taste buds, optimizing the ratios of sweet, bitter, sour, salty and umami. This can lead to fewer cravings and less desire for unhealthy foods. I have seen this occur with many of my clients.

Probiotics

I can't write a chapter about the power of our gastrointestinal tract without mentioning its main inhabitants. Currently, it is estimated that over 500 species of bacteria reside in the gut, and research has yet to identify them all.

Leon Chaitow, ND, DO, and Natasha Trenev explain some of the many benefits we acquire from the beneficial probiotic bacteria in our gut:[11]

Healthy microflora...
- manufacture specific B-vitamins
- help prevent cancer

- help deter the overgrowth of harmful microbes in our intestine by altering the pH of the region, depriving them of food, or producing antibacterial compounds against them
- favorably modify lipid markers
- have positive effects upon mood, including the alleviation of anxiety
- protect us from environmental exposures
- enhance our bowel function
- help regulate the recirculation of female estrogens

There are other benefits to balanced intestinal bacteria. For example, a study published in *Gut Pathogens* found that specific gut bacterial imbalances in infants from three weeks to one year old were linked to higher rates of obesity later in life:[12]

> *Recent research on obesity in humans and mice has demonstrated that the intestinal microflora can have an important influence on host energy balance ... In a study by Backhed et al., germfree mice colonized by Bacteroides thetaiotaomicron showed an increased weight gain and fat deposition as compared with germfree mice. The mechanism for this increased adiposity is at least partially the result of a microbial signal that suppresses the fasting-induced adipose factor (FIAF) of the host, resulting in increased production and storage of triglyceride derived fatty acids from the liver.*[12]

The fact that these little critters play a role in our metabolism has also been confirmed by the finding of different ratios of bacterial species in obese and diabetic adults versus healthy individuals. The ratios of bacterial species also influence mood and motor function. One study, reported in the *Proceedings of the National Academy of Sciences*, found that germ-free mice (animals bred to have no intestinal microflora) had different neurotransmitter patterns in their enteric and central nervous systems, which modified activity and anxiety-like behaviors.[13] This was in contrast to mice that were free of specific bacterial pathogens in the gut.

We all have a unique "bug blueprint" in the gut. As a result, we all have different metabolic and nutritional needs. Yet, thanks to the invention of quality probiotics (pro=for; biotic=life) and the ancient science of fermenting foods, we have the power to alter these little communities within our digestive tracts.

Taking a pill containing trillions of bugs doesn't necessarily repopulate the gut with healthy microbes and cancel out poor eating habits. Rather, it's been suggested that taking probiotics and eating a healthy diet help make the beneficial bacteria more welcome residents in our bodies and more able to provide their many health benefits. In fact, current research suggests that the beneficial actions that probiotics exert on our biochemistry may be more important than the actual number of organisms present. I have to agree. I have seen cases where the wrong probiotic for the wrong amount of time actually produced more gastrointestinal irritation in individuals. In these cases, my clients were blindly taking probiotics without making any dietary changes. They were also unaware of the quality and bacterial strain composition of their supplement. Therefore, getting assistance in finding the right probiotic for *you* is important.

The Bottom Line on Probiotic Supplements

I do recommend probiotics to most of my clients. Eating fermented foods such as organic coconut kefir, sauerkraut, miso, and tempeh is certainly a wise move, as they contain an abundance of probiotic strains. However, as an integrative doctor, I don't only use supplements to treat conditions; I also want to know why a person is off-balance. For example, if you aren't eating enough fiber (a.k.a. "bug food"), these little critters will never be properly balanced in your gut. I recommend different probiotics for different conditions. I also advise my clients to rotate strains and brands. I tend to use products that differ in their actions according to the specific strains that modulate inflammation, weight loss, and gastrointestinal motility, all selections being dependent on the person I am assisting.

A healthy diet and a good probiotic sometimes aren't enough to reverse a chronic condition, but they can be a good start! (Since this is too broad a topic to cover in this book, if you are interested in learning more about the critters that reside in our insides, please visit my database at dr-lobisco.com for more details.)

There are additional factors to consider for digestive and overall health. These include balancing digestive enzymes, removing small intestinal bowel overgrowth (a condition in which probiotics may actually be contraindicated!), balancing hormones, relieving oxidative stress, restoring proper neurotransmitter production, and balancing energy metabolism and inflammation. Furthermore, the whole body must be examined to find the underlying cause of one's problem. Below are some general considerations to keep your gut healthy, but remember that everyone has their own unique needs.

Tips for a Healthy Gastrointestinal Tract

1. Eat whole, unprocessed foods and include a rainbow of vegetables. The polyphenols and fiber in these plant foods feed healthy microflora. Also, eliminate possible food sensitivities, the most common being sugar, gluten, dairy, soy, corn, peanuts, and citrus fruits.
2. Start mending the gastrointestinal lining with nutritional herbs and supplements such as L-glutamine, zinc carnosine, deglycyrrhizinated licorice, aloe vera, marshmallow root, and chlorophyll. These products help repair the "leaks" in your

intestinal lining so that you don't keep dumping undigested particles into your system from your gastrointestinal tract.

3. Supplement with enzymes, as needed, to help you digest foods and prevent fermentation in the gut. Indications for digestive support include the following:

   a. Symptoms such as gas, reflux, and heartburn. A combination of betaine hydrochloric acid (HCL) and enzymes such as pepsin, proteases, lipases, amylases, cellulase, and invertase should be considered for complete digestive support.
   b. Aging, because we lose digestive prowess with time. In fact, around age 40, your ability to make the enzyme that digests proteins in the stomach begins to wane. Therefore, women and men entering mid-life may want to include betaine HCL in their digestive blend. HCL is contraindicated in anyone who has, or has had, an ulcer.
   c. Acne, which could indicate a need for betaine HCL, especially if it is located on the forehead.

4. Consider herbs and nutrients such as curcumin, ginger, licorice, methylsulfonylmethane (MSM), bromelain, quercetin, and other antioxidants to calm inflammation in the gut. Other helpful supplements include high-quality, purified krill oil, or 1000-2000 mg of DHA/EPA, found in a quality fish oil. For vegetarians, plant-based oils such as flax or hemp seed oil can be ingested. My personal favorite of these choices is krill oil, due to its additional antioxidant, brain, and eye benefits.

5. Use a probiotic that is appropriate for your type. For a wide range of my clients, I recommend rotating their probiotics every three to six months. This will ensure that they are getting a variety of organisms that support healthy digestion.

CHAPTER 6

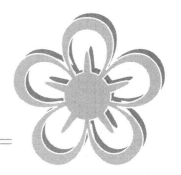

Healthy Body, Healthy Brain

In the previous chapter, I introduced the term "gut-brain." Many people are knowledgeable about the gut's role in digestion and elimination, but few are aware that it is responsible for producing most of the body's feel-good neurotransmitter, serotonin. Furthermore, the signaling molecules of other neurotransmitters, neuropeptides, and enkephalins are also made in the gut. These important chemical messengers assist with immune function, pain perception, and brain health.

This is why a healthy gut is so important for mood regulation and why it is the first organ system I discuss in this book. In any condition, it is important to find the cause, not just cover up the symptoms. Consequently, when dealing with any emotional or brain imbalance, it is important to look at the gut, the main source of the brain's signaling molecules. This gut-brain, termed the enteric nervous system (ENS), is very real and is a significant component of the mind-body connection.

The Conventional Approach to Depression

Depression is diagnosed based on criteria listed in the *Diagnostic and Statistical Manual of Mental Disorders*, now in its 5th edition (DSM-5). Symptoms of depression include:

- feelings of hopelessness, worthlessness, and/or guilt
- irritability
- low energy
- difficulty with brain functions such as memory, focus, and decision-making
- changes in sleeping patterns and/or appetite
- thoughts of suicide or attempts of suicide
- body aches and pains

According to the National Institute for Mental Health, there are several forms of depression:

Major depressive disorder, or major depression, is a form of depression that is severe enough to interfere with a person's ability to function, and lasts longer than two weeks. Most often, this form of depression is not limited to a single episode, but rather reoccurs throughout life. Along with the symptoms listed above, the sufferer often feels sad, anxious, or empty.

Dysthymic disorder, or dysthymia, is characterized by symptoms lasting two years or longer. It is not severe enough to disable a person, but does prevent normal functioning. People with this disorder can also periodically experience episodes of major depression.

Minor depression is related to a two-week or longer period of depression that is not severe enough to be classified as major depression.

There are other forms of depression that are atypical and have not yet been agreed upon for characterization:

- **Psychotic depression,** which is depression that occurs with psychotic episodes;
- **Postpartum depression,** which is a form of depression a new mother experiences after giving birth;
- **Seasonal affective disorder (SAD),** which is characterized by seasonal depression in the winter months that generally resolves in the spring; and
- **Bipolar disorder,** or **manic-depressive illness,** which is characterized by intense mood changes – from extreme highs (mania) to extreme lows (depression).

Women are twice as likely to suffer from depression as men. Furthermore, experiencing depression at a young age can have long-term health effects. In fact, children and adolescents who suffer from depression are more prone to severe illnesses later in life. Depression tends to be cyclical and can reoccur in many individuals, even if they are on medication.[1] In keeping with the theme of integrative medicine, all factors that influence mood and brain function should be investigated in a person suffering from depression. These include gastrointestinal health, hormonal imbalances, individual lifestyle characteristics, and genetics. By addressing lifestyle, diet, and other biochemical imbalances, rather than just manipulating neurotransmitter balance in the brain (the usual approach), a depressed individual can experience more lasting relief.

For example, social aspects should be considered when treating a person with depression. Those who are isolated have a higher incidence of mood imbalances. Feelings of being overwhelmed and overworked can affect our bodies' biochemistry in negative ways, and these changes tend to be more pronounced in those lacking support. In fact, social isolation is linked not only to a higher incidence of mood disorders but also to cardiovascular mortality. (See chapter 9 for more on the heart-connection discussion).

Therefore, a simple, yet effective solution to boost feel-good chemicals in your body is to reach out for support. The company of loved ones can stimulate an increase in dopamine and oxytocin – two feel-good brain chemicals that revive our brains. Unfortunately, in our dysfunctional society in which independence is so highly valued, many reach for something else for relief from their discomfort so they won't "be a burden" on others. This can lead to dependency and addiction; indeed, there is a link between depression and addictive patterns. This is because of the unmet need, in those who suffer emotionally, to feel comfort and safety from the company of others. Some seek to elicit this soothing response with certain foods, while others reach out for the numbing effect that a drink can offer. These practices can actually be a self-sabotaging (yet well-intentioned) attempt to cope.

A Pill for the Mentally Ill

Ten percent of the US population is currently taking antidepressant medications. Although medications can help get some people with depression back on track, using them without addressing the biological and lifestyle contributors to depression can result in the all-too-common "antidepressant shuffle." A 2010 meta-analysis published in JAMA concluded the following:

> The magnitude of benefit of antidepressant medication compared with placebo increases with severity of depression symptoms and may be minimal or nonexistent, on average, in patients with mild or moderate symptoms. For patients with very severe depression, the benefit of medications over placebo is substantial.[2]

This prompted an article released by *Psychology Today*, which featured a controversial opinion that one should avoid taking antidepressants.[3] The author quoted the meta-analysis as proof of the apparent ineffectiveness of these drugs in the majority of cases of non-severe depression. He also used it to debate the very premise of the neurotransmitter theory in which these drugs are aimed at manipulating brain chemistry. The author further ruffled conventional feathers when he cautioned against potential interactions with other drugs and discussed the harmful effects of society's "quick fix with a pill" mentality.

Still, because the conventional treatment for all types of depression is the use of antidepressants, it's important to understand the mechanism and theory behind them.

There are five main classes of antidepressant drugs:

- Selective Serotonin Reuptake Inhibitors (SSRIs): These medications block the brain's reuptake and breakdown of serotonin, the neurotransmitter in the brain that contributes to the sensation of well-being. The theory is that by keeping higher levels of this chemical in the brain for longer periods of time, depression will be alleviated. SSRIs are the most common class of antidepressants.
- Selective Serotonin and Norepinephrine Reuptake Inhibitors (SNRIs): These drugs increase the amount of both serotonin and norepinephrine in the brain, to improve mood, focus, and energy.
- Tricyclic Antidepressants (TCAs): An older group of drugs, TCAs are also used to treat obsessive-compulsive disorders, panic attacks, attention-deficit hyperactivity disorder (ADHD), and post-traumatic stress disorder (PTSD). These drugs also work by increasing serotonin and/or norepinephrine in the brain via a different mechanism than SNRIs.
- Monoamine Oxidase Inhibitors (MAOIs): These antidepressants increase serotonin, norepinephrine, dopamine, and other

monoamine neurotransmitters in the brain. They do this by inhibiting the enzyme monoamine oxidase, which normally recycles all of these neurotransmitters. MAOIs are the oldest form of antidepressants. They interact with many other drugs and foods, and have dangerous side effects due to *how* they impact this enzyme to increase neurotransmitter levels.
- Atypical antidepressants: This is varied group of medications that have different mechanisms of action to produce similar effects. For example, bupropion (Wellbutrin®) inhibits the reuptake of dopamine, serotonin and norepinephrine. Nefazodone (Serzone®) and venlafaxine (Effexor®) both increase the brain's levels of serotonin and norepinephrine. Trazodone (Desyrel®) is still not fully understood, but most likely works by inhibiting the reuptake of serotonin.

All of these drugs have a common effect. Regardless of their different mechanisms, they all affect the chemical messengers in the brain. Because SSRIs generally have fewer side effects than TCAs and MAOIs, they tend to be the first choice for treatment and are most often prescribed. For example, unlike MAOIs, SSRIs do not adversely interact with tyramine, a compound found in certain foods such as aged cheeses and red wine. They are also less apt to cause blood pressure fluctuations and heart arrhythmias.

However, SSRIs are not without risk. One caution regarding their use is the possibility of serotonergic syndrome, a condition that can feature high fever, seizure, and heart problems. Some other side effects and factors to consider with antidepressants include the following:

- They require time to build up in the body and become effective.
- Serious side effects and nutrient depletions can occur with each of these classes of drugs and should be supported.

- The most severe side effect, which has prompted mandatory governmental warnings, is a possible increase in suicidal thoughts.

  It's important to note that these medications can be lifesaving ... if properly prescribed.

In fact, I have seen cases where these medications have literally turned on the light switch in the brain of individuals who have been fighting the dark cloud of depression for years. These cases tend to have the following characteristics in common:

a. these individuals have a *true depletion* in that neurotransmitter, due to a lifestyle factor, environmental influence, or nutrient deficiency;

or...

b. they have *a genetic or structural issue* in the enzymes used to make or use these neurotransmitters.

In this way, the use of antidepressants may be necessary for a short period or indefinitely. In fact, they are one tool available that I discuss with my clients.

However, I am of the belief that, like most medications that are overprescribed for symptoms, antidepressants don't address all the root causes of the imbalance they are intended to correct. For example, SSRIs simply keep serotonin from being broken down or recycled by the brain; they don't make your body produce more serotonin. Unfortunately, most physicians aren't trained to look for which neurotransmitter deficiency causes which symptoms. Therefore, they are prescribing antidepressants in a trial-and-error fashion. In my opinion, messing with brain chemistry in this way is asking for trouble.

It's also important to remember that no pill in itself can fix a spiritual or emotional disconnect, unhealthy habits, or dysfunctional coping skill, though it may help a person make progress in these areas. These problems are also not helped merely by understanding *why* you are depressed. Speaking from the viewpoint of a mind-body-spirit healer, imbalances of this nature require support physically, emotionally, spiritually, and mentally in order to facilitate corrective action and results.

Why Drugs Are Missing the Mark

You've just read that one-tenth of Americans are currently taking an antidepressant; however, a 2008 meta-analysis in *PLoS Med* determined that antidepressants were no more likely to be effective than placebo for mild-to-moderate depression.[4] A long-term depression researcher, Eva Redei, discussed why these results made sense at the 2009 Neuroscience Conference in Chicago.[5]

According to findings from a rodent study, Redei and her colleagues felt that depression had been oversimplified and that drugs might be aimed at the wrong target. She challenged two strongly held beliefs about depression: that stressful life events or neurotransmitter imbalances of serotonin, norepinephrine, and dopamine trigger depression.

> *Redei found powerful molecular evidence that quashes the long-held dogma that stress is generally a major cause of depression … Redei found strong indications that depression actually begins further up in the chain of events in the brain. The biochemical events that ultimately result in depression actually start in the development and functioning of neurons.* "The medications have been focusing on the effect, not the cause," she said. "That's

why it takes so long for them to work and why they aren't effective for so many people."[5]

In other words, research suggests that the biochemical result – the *neurochemical effect* – of depression is way off. You might recall from Chapter 5 that over 70 percent of serotonin resides in your gut and that the gut's enteric nervous system interacts with many different enzymes and hormones to send feedback to the brain. This means that there's a pretty good chance that the foods that pass through the enteric system have an effect on our brain chemistry and resulting moods.

A recent Hungarian research article described the link between nutrition, mood, and food via digestion:

Local inflammation through the release of cytokines, neuropeptides and eicosanoids may also influence the function of the brain and of other organs. Role of metabolic burst due to inflammation represents a new aspect in both pathophysiology and treatment of the depression. Finally, an increasing number of clinical studies have shown that treating gastrointestinal inflammations with probiotics, vitamin B, D and omega 3 fatty acids, through attenuating proinflammatory stimuli to brain, may also improve depression symptoms and quality of life.[6]

The findings of this research suggest that gastrointestinal inflammation may relate to depression, and that treatment aimed to correct it may improve the efficiency of current treatments.

Many people are aware of a connection between feeling physical pain and feeling moody. As the body produces a defense response to the pain, these inflammatory pain mediators cause a decrease in feel-good neurotransmitters. Consequently, finding ways to decrease pain can impact how we feel, including our overall emotional balance.

This gut connection to pain, mood, and nutrition was demonstrated in a study[7] that reported on the mechanisms behind the ability of zinc (a mineral important for enzyme activation in blood sugar, immune function, and hormonal balance) to modulate the brain's perception of pain through its direct effect on this organ![7]

A More Integrated Approach to Treating Depression

Many physicians know that neurotransmitters can be affected by factors such as stress and emotional issues. However, few doctors are willing to look at how our brain can be affected by toxic chemicals, heavy metals, food sensitivities, nutritional deficiencies, infections, microbiota imbalances, and hormonal imbalances. Correcting these imbalances through nutrition, herbs, lifestyle, exercise, or appropriate medications can assist in addiction recovery, memory efficiency, and overall health.[8-9] I have seen remarkable changes in my clients' moods when they receive the nutritional and nutraceutical support based on their specific biochemical needs. In fact, this often enables them to make the emotional and lifestyle shifts that can alleviate their mood imbalances.

Physical conditions such as blood sugar imbalances, thyroid issues, adrenal insufficiency, or other endocrine dysfunctions can contribute to mood disorders through their interaction with brain signaling molecules. Hormonal imbalances, for example, can cause many changes in emotional status because hormones play an important role as chemical messengers in the body and can affect the brain's levels of neurotransmitters.[10] By addressing underlying hormonal issues and supporting organ or gland dysfunction with nutrition, medicinal essential oils and herbals, many women in my clinic have noticed significant changes in their emotional well-being.

Depression can also result from decreased blood oxygenation[11] to the brain through various causes. In addition, brain health can be altered by exposure to chemicals and toxins.[12-14] Both, in turn, can cause imbalances in brain chemistry and multiple negative health effects. Some therapeutic-grade essential oils, such as cedarwood,[15-18] neroli,[19-20] and lavender,[21-25] have been shown to assist with mood and support neural health. Due to the fact that they contain a variety of chemical constituents, including sesquiterpenes,[26-31] these, and other essential oils, are effective in modulating many pathways in the body,[32-35] including those involved in mood regulation.

Eating for mental health is as much of a commitment as is eating for a healthy body. In order for the body to produce mind-boosting chemicals, we need to take in cofactors such as zinc, B vitamins, magnesium, and vitamin C[36] on a daily basis.

If the above considerations don't effectively eliminate mood imbalances, some people can benefit from specialized testing to determine their utilization of various neurotransmitters. This specific testing, along with an assessment for nutrient deficiencies, provides specifications for a comprehensive plan that helps modulate levels of neurotransmitters and helps the body more effectively make its own.

Another key tool in stabilizing mood is mind-body medicine.[37] People today are overworked, over-stressed, and tend to devalue themselves. Mindfulness and the willingness to feel one's emotions, rather than suppress them, can be of great value to a person searching for balance. There are also various individualized relaxation and stress-reducing techniques I implement in my practice that help people deal with everyday stressors or relationship issues. These include Emotional Freedom Technique (EFT)[38], Heart Coherence, and meditation guidance.

Additionally, "natural buffers" exist that support the body through stressful transition periods. If a client wishes to explore various modalities, we will work to find the optimal herbal or nutritional program for our purposes. A standardized preparation of the herb, St. John's wort,[39] is helpful to some for mild-to-moderate depression, and has been shown to be just as effective for mild depression as antidepressant drug therapy.[8] It reacts, however, with many medications, thus its use should be monitored by a healthcare professional.

S-adenosylmethionine (SAMe), 5-hydroxytryptophan (5-HTP), fish oils, and B vitamins[36,39] can also help boost one's mood, depending on which symptoms and deficiencies a person is exhibiting. The most important factor is *individualization* of approach, based on the cause of the depression and the region of the brain that is producing depressive symptoms.

Looking into the Brain

Addressing the factors contributing to depression, *as well as* the location in the brain, is important in providing an optimized plan for mood and emotional well-being. Discovering the area of the brain that is most affected will determine when, how, and what supplements will produce the best results.

In my practice, I use a combination of case history, information about a client's cognition, testing, and questionnaires. Specifically, I give my clients a "brain balance" questionnaire adapted from Dr. Amen's work.[9] This questionnaire enables me to not only identify areas of the brain that are out of balance, but also to track progress in symptom relief. The side effect of a stabilized brain is better balance in overall health. After all, a healthy brain modulates all healthy behaviors!

When clients become aware of the five main parts of the brain, their functions, and what contributes to imbalances, they gain an understanding of why certain patterns are hard to break. This is important in healing the self-deprecation that often accompanies mood imbalances. For instance, when an imbalance in one or more areas becomes hardwired as a habitual pattern, what can appear as self-sabotaging behavior can be viewed more as a dysfunctional brain process than a judgment of one's self-worth.

For clinicians, this information can prove essential in determining the correct support. This can make the difference between mood improvement and continued mood aggravations. For example, someone can be anxious because of an overactive stress response in one region of the brain or because of an underactive calming response in another location. Hence, the nutritional or medicinal interventions will be different, depending on which area is most affected.

To help you understand the difference between the functions of various parts of the brain, I have provided a list below of the functions of the five most common areas of the brain and some balancing tips and nutrients that I consider, based on an individual's unique makeup and symptom picture.

The following information is adapted from Dr. Amen's work:[9]

I. Deep Limbic System Functions

The deep limbic system is a set of brain structures that regulate a variety of functions. These areas act mostly to regulate the drive to meet our basic needs (safety, sex, connection, and appetite). It functions to…

- provide emotional tone of the mind by…
  - affecting memory storage and emotional cues
  - acting as a filter for external events by providing the "fight and flight" response and setting the level of importance to them
- modulate motivation
- control appetite and sleep cycles
- promote bonding and modulate libido (sex drive)
- directly process olfaction (sense of smell)

Deep Limbic System Balancing Tips

- Rid your brain of what Dr. Amen terms "the ANTs" (Autonomic Negative Thoughts).
    - ANTs trump mood by repeating cynical, gloomy, or self-deprecating thoughts.
    - You can train yourself to recognize a thought as an "ANT" versus a truth statement, and stomp on the thought by replacing it with a positive one.
- Try the three interventions below to decrease the burden on the brain of the stress response and to evoke the hormone, oxytocin. This will modulate the negative thoughts and promote healing.
    - Surround yourself with positive people and build people skills to enhance connection to others. Bonding with others boosts immunity and well-being, whereas staying in isolation promotes stress and fear.
    - Value and promote physical contact.
    - Surround yourself with appealing scents, which activate olfaction through the diffusion of therapeutic essential oils.
- Build a library of wonderful memories by participating more in your own life.
    - Consider mingling with others or enjoying your own time without guilt. Positive experiences in your hippocampus – the memory center – will accumulate until they eventually trump the negative ANTS that attack your mood!
- Exercise, for a lot of reasons.
    - Exercise boosts endorphins, the body's own and free feel-good chemicals. (Healthy diets, including organic protein sources and amino acid protein shakes, will add a power punch to this effect.)
    - Exercise also boosts serotonin, dopamine, and other feel-good brain and heart chemicals.

- Exercise improves blood sugar modulation, which affects mood stabilization.
- Exercise cleanses your lymph system, which filters blood and helps your body eliminate toxins more effectively. A toxic body makes for a toxic mind.

Nutrients for Balancing & Calming the Deep Limbic System

- Fish oil
- Minerals
- L-tyrosine (an amino acid that supports the thyroid, calms a stressed-out brain, and acts as a precursor to dopamine)
- L-phenylalanine (an essential amino acid that assists in the production of endorphins and other neurotransmitters)
- N-acetylcysteine (NAC) (an antioxidant precursor which can also be used to calm the brain by recycling the excitatory chemical, glutamate; it may also help reduce emotional food or substance cravings)
- 5-HTP or gamma-aminobutyric acid (GABA) (supplements that can be used to balance serotonin or endogenous GABA as needed)

II. Basal Ganglia System Functions

This system is the integrator of feelings and the execution of movement. Specifically, these functions include…

- assistance with fine motor behavior
- acting as a "stop command" to suppress unwanted motor behaviors such as tremors
- regulating the body's tone at rest
- impacting the level of emotional reactions, including anxiety
- enhancing motivation
- mediating feelings of pleasure and ecstasy

Tips for Balancing the Basal Ganglia System

For most people with an overactive basal ganglia system, the following activities can be balancing and calming. These exercises can be especially helpful to those who are anxious or have anxious depression. They can assist in breaking the cycle of negative, fear-provoking, future predictions:

- Use guided imagery and meditation.
    - CDs or iTunes apps are available from many self-help or meditative gurus. Find one that soothes you.
- Practice diaphragmatic breathing.
    - Most people's shallow breathing triggers more anxiety. This causes a decrease in the flow of vital oxygen to important organs and will result in activating the reactionary side of the nervous system response.
    - Breathing deeply into your abdomen will increase "vagal tone." The vagus nerve signals our nervous system to a "rest and digest response," which will result in improved oxygenation, calmness, and cleansing.
- Mentally stomp on those negative fortune-telling ANTs. This is in order to stop runaway anxious thoughts that can lead to further panic, isolation, and conflict avoidance.
- Enlist a group of people who can support you. Include yourself! Find someone you respect and use that person's objective feedback to find positive ways to deal with uncomfortable situations rather than to avoid them.
- Essential oils help this region of the brain as well.
    - Surround yourself with scents that are calming to the brain, especially the oils of chamomile and lavender.
- Avoid stimulants or alcohol, which increase anxiety, directly or paradoxically, in your system.

Nutrients for Supporting the Basal Ganglia System

- L-tyrosine, as needed, for thyroid and stress support
- Minerals (especially magnesium), to help calm the brain and body
- B vitamins (various B vitamins assist with hormonal and neurotransmitter support, especially B6, an important cofactor in neurotransmitter production)
- Adrenal gland support
  - It is essential to support your stress response when modulating brain function. This can be done partly by supporting the adrenal glands, which are responsible for the release of stress hormones cortisol, adrenaline (epinephrine), and noradrenaline (norepinephrine). Herbal supplements, such as *Withania somnifera*, known as ashwagandha or Indian ginseng, can modulate GABA, a calming neurotransmitter, and provide support for the stress response.
  - Nutrients such as vitamin B6, vitamin B5, vitamin C, and various essential minerals can be incorporated to nourish the adrenal glands and to mitigate the stress response.
- Individualized neurotransmitter support through GABA, SAMe, or NAC, as needed

III. Prefrontal Cortex (PFC) Functions

Think of this region as the "executive" of tasks. A fully-functioning PFC will positively affect the following functions and serve as the key player in self-monitoring and self-supervision:

- attention span
- perseverance
- judgment

- impulse control
- organization
- problem-solving
- critical thinking
- forward-thinking and learning from experience
- ability to feel and express emotions appropriately (empathy)
- interaction with the limbic system (emotional center) to translate stressors and provide input about them

Prefrontal Cortex (PFC) Balancing Exercises

- Try the One-Page Miracle: Write down all your goals on one page in order to stimulate your brain's executive functioning. This will also help shift your focus in a positive direction.
- Keep your mind focused on positive outcomes instead of negative outcomes. This will keep your emotional tone more rational, and ignite the PFC.
- Include self-care and joy in your life in order to re-ignite a sense of purpose and to give your brain some downtime to recharge it's "productivity" mindset
- Get organized! Free your brain of clutter by writing "to-do" lists. Here are some helpful hints:
    - Use a scheduler or write down tasks on a calendar, and create check-lists of what you want to accomplish (sanely) that day.
    - Make sure you give yourself some wiggle room so that you don't feel overwhelmed when looking at your list. This would defeat the purpose! Consider making three columns for the following categories:
        1. Three major tasks that must be accomplished that day
        2. Goals you'd like to complete within the week but that aren't pressing today

3. Long-term projects or goals that will become a priority in time and which should be worked on periodically to avoid panic
- Get biofeedback training with a certified specialist who can help retrain your brain.
- Hire a coach to help call you out on negative procrastination patterns and assist you in creating that "to-do" list.
- Cut out the over-stimulation – stop yelling, speak gently, take some stillness and "quiet time" to retune with your own innate wisdom. Constant background noise is a stimulus that your nervous system has to work to drown out, and creates additional strain and stress. If you need background noise, consider listening to music that relaxes the brain and induces positive neural impulses, such as classical music, especially Mozart.

Nutrients for Supporting the Prefrontal Cortex

- Fish oil, to calm inflammation and support transmission between neurons.
- L-tyrosine, L-phenylalanine, and L-Dopa, for their dopamine and thyroid-supporting functions
- Adrenal support and minerals that calm the limbic system and basal ganglia, in order to turn on the PFC
- Antioxidants that contain the constituents OPCs (oligomeric proanthocyanidins)
- Green tea
- 5-HTP can help an overactive and anxious PFC, whereas dopamine precursors can be used to stimulate an underactive and depressed PFC

IV. Functions of the Cingulate Gyrus

Think of the cingulate gyrus as your brain's gear shifter between its two hemispheres. A healthy cingulate system is essential to your ability to flow and transition with life. Besides helping to modulate involuntary processes and sensations, it is important for...

- shifting of attention from one task to the next
- cognitive flexibility, which allows different parts of the brain to be incorporated for a particular task, such as your creative brain hemisphere with your logical hemisphere
- general adaptability and in tasks such as the following:
  - movement from idea to idea
  - ability to "go with the flow" with schedule shifts
  - ability to cooperate in a team and see others' options

Cingulate System Balancing Exercises

- Build the muscles in your gear shifter when you notice you're stuck on an idea, thought, or task.
  - In this instance, distract yourself from the repetitive thought pattern, shift your focus, and return to the problem later with a fresh perspective.
  - Write out different options from what you've been considering, in order to gain a new perspective.
  - If you tend to be logical, consider drawing a diagram to ignite your creative brain. If you tend to be more artistic and have problems with logic, try to incorporate more logic by using lists and computations of solutions.
- Press the pause button when you are asked a question, and take advantage of others' support in considering alternative responses. Many people with an overactive cingulate system tend to respond in a knee-jerk fashion and can appear

"stubborn." Think before saying "no" or "yes" to a common request. This will help you gain more access to all areas of your brain.
    - Seek counsel from people you respect when weighing options, to obtain a fresh viewpoint.
- Use the serenity prayer if you are having a hard time turning over damaging or unhelpful thoughts or patterns. Here is the prayer with an explanation:
    - "God (or whoever/whatever you consider to be a higher power), grant me the serenity to accept the things I cannot change (get out of this negative pattern), courage to change the things I can (try a new perspective), and wisdom to know the difference (let go of controlling outcomes, but focus on your contribution).
- Move your body!
    - Exercise and movement will literally bring more cerebral blood flow to all areas of your brain and get you "out of your head."

Nutrients for Supporting the Cingulate System

- According to your symptoms, minerals, vitamins, and amino acids can be used to support various neurotransmitters; e.g., 5-HTP, L-tryptophan, and serotonin precursors, all used with appropriate supervision
- Adrenal nutrition, such as was mentioned in the previous brain sections
- Munch on healthy carbs
    - The key is to include healthy carbohydrates that are slow-burning for this area of the brain. Examples include root vegetables like carrots, sweet potatoes or yams, or slow-cooked gluten-free grains, such as rice and quinoa. These foods will assist in moving tryptophan past the blood-brain

barrier for serotonin production. Therefore, for example, Paleolithic and high-protein diets won't support rebalancing the cingulate system.
- o Remember, moderation is the key. Too much sugar will promote anxiety, so make sure you balance with protein and don't "supersize."

V. Functions of the Temporal Lobe

Your temporal lobe has various roles that span from translating sense perception and the deciphering of emotions, to the storage of memories. (It is the home of the famous hippocampus). Some of the functions of this lobe include...

- language comprehension
    - o visual and auditory learning and processing
    - o decoding of vocal cues and recognition of facial expressions
    - o retrieval of words and visual memories
- memory operations and storage related to...
    - o intermediate-term memory
    - o long-term memory
    - o complex memories
- emotional stability

Temporal Lobe Balancing Exercises

- Balance the deep limbic system to modulate emotions by using the tips in that section. Memory storage and retrieval are colored by the emotional tone of the limbic brain; therefore, stress really *can* make you "stupid"!
- Bring music to your life. Use these activities to help fire the temporal lobe:
    - o Sing a song or hum

- - Repeat a tone; Dr. Amen suggests the following:
    - "Ahhh" for evoking a relaxation response
    - "Ee" or "ay" to help concentration, release pain/anger
    - "Oh" or "om" to relax muscle tension
  - Listen to classical music or play a musical instrument you enjoy
  - Move to rhythm – chanting, dancing, and/or singing
- Getting a full night's sleep will increase oxygenation and help balance mood. Dr. Amen points out how continually getting less than six hours of sleep has been shown to cause decreased perfusion to the brain.

Nutrients to Consider for the Temporal Lobe

- GABA and/or magnesium, to relieve anxiety (that prevents focus) and help calm the brain
- Phosphatidylserine and phosphatidylcholine, important components of brain neurons, to help calm the brain, stabilize mood, and support memory

The Link for All Brain Functions

After reviewing a client's brain questionnaire, I begin implementing the various suggestions discussed above based on the individual's specific brain's needs. I also select appropriate essential oils to further support bringing one's brain back in balance. Essential oils, not to be confused with essential fatty acids, are the life-blood of the plant from which they're derived. They are distilled from various parts of a plant, using a special process that keeps all of the constituents intact. Essential oils differ from dried herbs, in which the essential oil has usually been processed out. Both herbs and essential oils hold a very special place in Nature's pharmacy.

Due to the aromatic constituents in essential oils, they can more powerfully affect the brain as compared to dried herbs and, when inhaled, can go directly to the limbic and emotional centers.[40-45] This inhalation creates harmony and balance while easing tension throughout the body. As mentioned, calming the emotional tone will affect feedback to all areas of our elegant cerebral cortex, making all of these regions work more effectively. I've provided a brief summary below of the various oils I've found most useful in my practice.

Before you read on, it's important that I make two very important **disclaimers:**

1. In listing all of the constituents of an essential oil, my purpose is to portray the synergism of the whole plant oil. By keeping the integrity of all of its properties intact, these therapeutic oils contain all the necessary ingredients for whatever is needed in the body. For example, if a person has a respiratory infection, the ketones, alcohols, and phenols will exert the most powerful effect *at that time for that individual.* If high blood pressure is an issue, the sesquiterpenes and calming esters will override the stimulating phenols and oxides to calm this same system.[43,45]

This is why I tell my clients that the oils have "a mind of their own." It's the brilliance of Mother Nature's recipes! As an analogy, compare it to including the (organic, gluten-free) cookie with its chocolate chips, rather than isolating out the chips. Eating only the chips would produce a more intense caffeine-like effect.

2. This information is applicable *only* for therapeutic, Grade A (genuine) essential oils. This information does *not* apply to essential oils that have not been assessed for quality control or regulation in the United States. For example, oils labeled as "100% pure" need only contain 5 percent of the actual oil; the

rest of the bottle may contain fillers or toxic ingredients that could cause harm. [40-42]

This is why I stick with essential oils that I have researched and whose quality I am certain about. Among my top favorite brands is Young Living Essential Oils. In fact, I was a distributor of these oils before I became a naturopathic doctor. After experiencing their healing power first-hand, I began my search for more integrative medical training.

As always, remember that all information in this book is meant to empower you with knowledge to make your own decisions and is *not* intended to diagnose, treat, or prescribe for any illness.

All of the oils listed below can be applied topically or inhaled for enhancing the mood. Ingesting oils or using them rectally is usually reserved for sickness, including respiratory infections.[40-43] (Ingesting oils usually requires working with a qualified practitioner.) It's best to start by applying one to two drops on the bottom of the feet. This is because the feet have the largest pores for absorption compared to the rest of the body, and are not as likely as other areas to develop a skin rash. The most benefit comes from placing a few drops of your favorite oil on your hands and inhaling the scent whenever you feel anxious or sad. You can also purchase a cold-air diffuser, which will allow you to enjoy the aroma throughout the room.

Lavender

Known as the "universal oil," lavender is probably the most well-known essential oil in modern times. Many people are familiar with its calming and relaxing fragrance. With its wide array of constituents, this gentle oil is safe for everyone and is known to balance the body and work wherever in the body there is need. There is a famous catch phrase in aromatherapy: "When in doubt, use lavender!"

However, few people in the United States are aware that lavender is a powerful therapeutic oil that contains over 300 medicinal constituents when properly distilled.

In 1910, Dr. Rene-Maurice Gattefosse, a French chemist, discovered lavender's skin regenerating properties during World War I.[46] When his severely burned arm healed without a scar, Dr. Gattefosse began studying the constituents of essentials oils and instigated the re-dissemination of modern-day medical aromatherapy knowledge.[47] As a result of his lab discovery, lavender is still listed in the British Pharmacopoeia for its healing properties in the skin.

I have also had great success in my practice using lavender for hormonal issues, skin problems, sleep disturbances, "nervous stomach," mood support, and restlessness.[21-23, 25, 48-49]

Valerian

Valerian has been clinically investigated for over thirty years and, according to the German Commission E, it's an effective treatment for restlessness and sleep disturbances.[50-53] Some studies have even favorably compared the effectiveness of valerian root to pharmaceutical sleep aids.[50]

Scientists believe that the sedative action of valerian may be due to its effect on the neurotransmitter gamma aminobutyric acid (GABA) in the brain.[50-53] However, several studies have exhibited that valerian constituents may also influence other receptors that effect brain activity, including serotonin[54] and adenosine.[55] A 2003 study in *American Physician* stated the following on the mechanism of valerian:

> The chemical composition of valerian includes sesquiterpenes of the volatile oil (including valeric acid), iridoids (valepotriates), alkaloids, furanofuran lignans, and free amino acids such as γ-aminobutyric acid (GABA), tyrosine, arginine, and glutamine. Although the sesquiterpene components of the volatile oil are believed to be responsible for most of valerian's biologic effects, it is likely that all of the active constituents of valerian act in a synergistic manner to produce a

> *clinical response. Research into physiologic activity of individual components has demonstrated direct sedative effects (valepotriates, valeric acid) and interaction with neurotransmitters such as GABA (valeric acid and unknown fractions).*[56]

Therefore, I've suggested the use of valerian to help in situations where calming the nervous system will be beneficial in the alleviation of symptoms related to sleep disturbances, nervous indigestion, headaches, restlessness, and nervous tension.[51-52] I've found that this oil can be very supportive when a person has a temporal lobe imbalance and resultant mood symptoms as well. In fact, a 2014 observation study demonstrated improvement in restlessness and concentration in 164 primary school children by using a combination of valerian root and lemon balm.[57]

Neroli
The essential oil of neroli, from the Rutaceae family, is another oil which has been shown to have calming effects on the brain.[58-60] Some studies have demonstrated its influence on serotonin[58] and GABA,[59] which may relate to this relaxation response. One study demonstrated its positive effects on menopausal symptoms, stress, and estrogen in postmenopausal women.[20] It has also been shown to support the immune system and act as a strong antioxidant.[61-62] One rodent study suggests that neroli may assist with inflammation in the colon, which may make neroli helpful for supporting gut-brain communication.[63]

There are many other essential oils which can support the brain. I have highlighted three for simplicity only. If you are interested in learning more about these essential oils and other wellness uses, please visit my essential oils database on my website, dr-lobisco.com

Remember, You're Not in This Alone

As part of a holistic approach to wellness, we know that emotions affect every aspect of a person's life, including physical well-being, spirituality, and relationships with others. In today's world, it is unfortunately very common to feel alone and isolated. Depression can make you feel even more isolated, which only compounds the intensity of these sometimes overwhelming feelings. *Reaching out for support is a sign of strength and empowerment!*

If you want a holistic approach to your health, it's important to find a practitioner who is trained in both conventional and holistic approaches. It is optimal to search for a practitioner who will look for specific nutrient deficiencies and correct any imbalances, and/or have the means to minimize side effects when a medication is being used. Naturopathic and functional medicine doctors are examples of such professionals. They have the training and ability to work comprehensively with clients, addressing their unique physiology and root causes of symptoms, from physical to emotional and spiritual.

Your physician and holistic health practitioner should ideally work together to get to the bottom of your mood disturbances, so that you can live a healthy, happier life.

CHAPTER 7

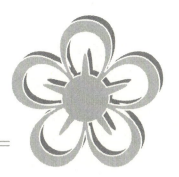

Finding Hormonal Harmony

H ormones are chemical messengers that play an intricate role in overall health. They help maintain metabolism at the cellular level, as well as modulate blood sugar, inflammation, immunity, and sexual organ function. The most well-known hormones – the reproductive hormones – are produced within the sex glands themselves, as well as in the adrenals, a pair of glands located on top of the kidneys. However, hormones are so vital for biochemical balance that they are manufactured throughout the entire body.[1-2] For example, did you know the heart produces hormones that balance various systems, including immunity?[3]

Because of their far-reaching effects at the smallest of doses, hormonal output is tightly controlled by complex feedback systems. The hypothalamus in the brain is the main regulator of most hormonal activity. Specifically, it monitors the amount of hormones in the blood. If levels drop too low, the hypothalamus will release a signal to the pituitary gland. Once the pituitary gland receives this signal, it will release a stimulatory signal to a target organ to increase hormonal output. After this hormone has attained a sufficient level, the hypothalamus releases an inhibitory signal to the pituitary to stop its stimulatory signaling to the target organ. As a result, production of this hormone takes a break.[1-2]

Due to the fact that hormones are very powerful, a spike or a drop in these chemicals, even in minute degrees, can have multidimensional effects. This means that when our hormones and their control mechanisms are optimally balanced, our bodies respond appropriately to physical and emotional stressors. However, if something causes an imbalance in their production or in these feedback loops, uncomfortable and wide-ranging symptoms can result. Examples include weight gain,[4-5] blood sugar fluctuations,[6-7] immune problems,[8] reproductive imbalances,[9] and mood changes.[9-10] Furthermore, any suboptimal hormone level can affect a variety of organs all at once!

Hormones Off Balance

The impact of hormonal balance is so far-reaching that an imbalance in one hormone also affects the levels of other hormones, triggering a cascade of symptoms.[1-10] This is especially true for the sex hormones DHEA, estrogen, progesterone, and testosterone. For this reason alone, it is important to determine the root cause of any hormonal dysfunction, rather than to simply treat the symptoms, even with "safe," natural methods. As an example, variations in levels of estrogen, testosterone, and insulin can influence production of the proteins sex-hormone-binding globulin and thyroid-binding globulin, produced mostly in the liver. Among other effects, this can reduce thyroid hormone availability.[11-13] The precursor to the active hormone may be present and at a normal level in the blood, but conversion to the active hormone could be "stuck in a rut." The result can be *symptoms of deficiency, even when there isn't one.*

The Importance of Testing & the Caveats

Therefore, when putting something as powerful as a hormone in your body, it is a good idea to test and monitor its level. This can be done with the help of a knowledgeable naturopathic or functional medicine practitioner. It is best to select a healthcare provider who has an understanding of both the shortcomings and usefulness of the different methods of measuring hormones, as well as how to interpret them for your specific needs.

Below is a summary list of laboratory tests to consider with your doctor when checking for hormonal imbalances:

A. A full thyroid panel. Many doctors measure only thyroid-stimulating hormone (TSH), to check thyroid function. TSH alone is not sufficient to measure thyroid hormone status, since it only measures the pituitary's stimulation of the thyroid gland. This leaves many hypothyroid sufferers undertreated and underdiagnosed.[14]

Instead, I recommend that my clients request a measurement of available thyroid hormone in its free form, i.e., FT3 and FT4. Furthermore, I like to obtain specific antibody tests, including TPO (thyroid peroxidase) and TgAb (thyroglobulin antibody), to help rule out autoimmune causes of thyroid imbalances. I also suggest an ultrasound to monitor for any changes in the thyroid tissue from an experienced physician.[15]

B. Salivary and serum hormonal panels including: estrogens, progesterone, testosterone, sex hormone-binding globulin (SHBG), and a cortisol/DHEA ratio (saliva). DHEA, or dehydroepiandrosterone, is the precursor hormone for many sex hormones, and can be depleted from excess stress.[16]

C. Salivary cortisol and urinary neurotransmitter balances, to evaluate total adrenal health. (See caveats, below)

Other factors involved in hormonal production, modulation, and feedback should also be tested. These include...

1. Blood sugar markers: Glucose, insulin, and hemoglobin A1c (which reflects glucose levels over a 3-month period)
2. Lipid panels for heart disease risk: Cholesterol, HDL-C, LDL-C, lipoprotein particle size (using a NMR panel), triglycerides, apolipoproteins (ApoA1 and ApoB), homocysteine, and hsCRP
3. Nutritional assessments for vitamin and mineral deficiencies
4. Immune and inflammatory measurements, such as testing for Lyme disease, latent or stealth infections (such as EBV, CMV, or other viruses), and inflammatory signaling markers (such as cytokines)
5. Intestinal health markers, which may include food sensitivity panels (e.g., from Cyrex or ALCAT Labs), intestinal permeability markers (e.g., Cyrex or Dunwoody Labs), microbiome diversity tests, and stool analysis for microbes and parasites
6. Testing for toxic elements, including heavy metals (e.g., from Genova Diagnostics or Doctor's Data)

When testing and assessing the results of your lab tests, consider the following caveats:

1. Serum labs mostly measure *bound* hormones (i.e., hormones held in reserve) and don't assess for how they're utilized in the body. Furthermore, they aren't accounting for metabolized hormones or the amount concentrated in tissues or fat reserve.
2. The feedback mechanisms for estrogen production differ with age. In premenopausal women, sex hormone production occurs mostly in the ovaries. In postmenopausal women, estrogen is formed in peripheral tissue and is more dependent on adrenal production of precursor hormones. Therefore, assessing adrenal function is an additional factor to consider.[17]

3. When evaluating adrenal function, most integrative doctors use salivary testing of cortisol. However, salivary cortisol and hormonal salivary panels, in general, don't account for all hormone metabolites, their excretion rate, or storage of the hormones in distant sites.
    - For example, cortisol can break down to cortolones and cortols, based on favored enzyme pathways. These are rarely measured.[18]
    - Thus, to get the most complete picture of your adrenal health, it is helpful to include measurements of urinary metabolites of the stress hormones, adrenaline and noradrenaline, along with salivary cortisol levels.
4. The health of a woman's liver or gut, and genetic influences on a woman's ability to metabolize hormones (which varies greatly among women) can all impact how a hormone is used in the body.[19-20] Making sure at the start that your digestive tract is in good shape is a good way to ensure that hormones will be utilized and excreted (see chapter 5). Also consider the following individual measurements:
    - A test that measures the ratio of 2/16 estrogen metabolites in the body[21-23]
    - Testing for individual variations in DNA sequences within the genes controlling enzymes that break down hormones, termed single nucleotide polymorphisms (SNPs). These markers can provide information on how well a woman can metabolize a suggested hormonal therapy.[24-25]

As you can see, a thorough evaluation for any hormonal imbalance includes a whole-body approach. All of the above factors, along with proper timing of tests, can guide your practitioner's recommendations regarding the appropriate use and form of a hormone (such as a cream or pill), hormone dosage, or the possibility of herbal therapies.

Moreover, nutrient deficiencies,[26] stress, genetic predisposition, and lifestyle patterns all have an impact on the effects of hormonal therapy, so should be considered during hormonal support.

These considerations can appear daunting. This is why I suggest a consultation with an integrative or functional medical practitioner who can evaluate the cause of the problem and suggest an individualized treatment plan.

Now, we are going to highlight some specific hormonal imbalances and symptom pictures that can be used in combination with laboratory findings to arrive at solutions.

The Thyroid Connection

Thyroid problems are among the most common causes of hormonal disorders in the United States.[27] Thyroid hormones have an important role in a variety of body regulatory processes, such as carbohydrate, protein and fat metabolism, vitamin utilization, mitochondrial function and energy production, digestion, muscle and nerve activity, blood flow, oxygen utilization, hormonal balance, and overall metabolism.[27-29]

Due to the fact that thyroid hormone interacts with so many biochemical messengers, including brain neurotransmitters, suboptimal thyroid function can produce a myriad physical and emotional issues. Any of the symptoms below may prompt you to consider a full thyroid evaluation as described above:

- dry skin and hair
- weight gain
- physical weakness
- muscle cramps
- decreased libido
- brain fog
- menstrual irregularities

- fatigue
- yellowed skin tone (thyroid hormone plays a role in the conversion of beta carotene to vitamin A in the liver; therefore, reduced conversion causes beta carotene to accumulate in the skin)
- emotional imbalances such as depressive symptoms, irritability, and anxiety[27-29]

Stressed-Out Hormones

Most people have heard of cortisol, a stress hormone produced by the adrenal glands. It functions to ignite the survival response when we're faced with a threat. In a stressful situation, precursor hormones convert to cortisol instead of sex hormones, thereby affecting the levels of estrogen, testosterone, or progesterone. Survival and reproduction are mutually exclusive. Although important in the short term, excessive cortisol over time can cause long-term hormonal imbalances. In turn, these can lead to a vast array of symptoms, including weight changes, mood swings, menstrual cycle disturbances, food cravings, and blood sugar imbalances.[30-33]

Looking at it another way, chronic stress keeps the car on the road, but puts it in park. This creates a vicious cycle, in which extra cortisol is made to compensate for the low energy resulting from impaired thyroid hormone activation. This effect is compounded by the release of other stress-signaling molecules in the adrenal gland, i.e., adrenaline and noradrenaline, which can perpetuate this prolonged stress response.[34]

This imbalance in chemicals has an initial excitatory effect on the brain, making one feel irritable, anxious, and fatigued (a.k.a. "wired and tired"). Eventually, the adrenal glands can't keep up with the demand, and reduced amounts of adrenaline, noradrenaline, mineralocorticoids, and cortisol result. This end stage of "adrenal fatigue" can include debilitating exhaustion, depression, fluid retention, and chronic immune disorders.

Cortisol also has an impact on immune function and profound systemic effects. For example, in the short term, cortisol acts to turn down the dial on the immune system, suppressing the inflammatory response. This is productive during those times when you need greater energy reserves to survive, or when you have had an accident and your body needs to "cool down." However, long-term stress and suppression of the immune system can make you more prone to illness and delayed healing.[34-35] When cortisol is depleted, uncontrolled inflammation and pain can result. (Prednisone and steroids are medications that mimic the effects of cortisol and are often used to suppress pain and inflammation. Side effects of these drugs can include immune suppression, bone loss, fluid retention, and weight gain.)

High amounts of cortisol during a prolonged stress response can also cause problems with blood sugar. This is because raised levels of cortisol signal your pancreas to increase its production of the hormone, insulin.[30,37] Over time, this increased demand can overload the pancreas and cause insulin resistance, which interferes with the proper uptake of glucose and other essential nutrients into the cells. The body may have plenty of fuel in this situation, but it will not absorb it correctly, thus be starved for nutrition in the presence of an adequate food supply. The result can be intense food cravings, digestive issues, increased fat storage, and high levels of triglycerides in the bloodstream. Weight gain and various hormonal symptoms can also intensify, as increasing insulin resistance also dysregulates other hormonal and appetite-inhibiting signals, such as leptin.

The downstream effects of chronic stress on the body are summarized below:

- Gastrointestinal issues, specifically decreased absorption and resultant inflammation in the gut. This causes the enteric nervous system region of the intestine, where most of your neurotransmitters are formed, to produce less calming serotonin (see chapter 5).

- Hormonal imbalances due to stress hormones being made from precursor hormones that would otherwise go toward the production of sex hormones.
- Weight gain, as the body stores fuel for later use, and from blood sugar imbalances due to insulin resistance.
- Mood and memory disturbances due to changes in brain biochemistry.
- Other conditions that can result from stress-induced nutritional deficiencies, chronic suppression of inflammation, and immune imbalances.[30-37]

More On the "Numbing" Effects of Stress

We discussed how stress can affect your brain biochemistry and mood. Stress can also affect your memory, to the point of making you feel "stupid."[38-41] There are a few reasons for this…

First, chronic stress depletes the body of thyroid, estrogen, and progesterone, all of which interact with other brain signals. Second, it shuts down digestion and reduces the gut's production of the calming neurotransmitter, serotonin. The excitatory stress hormones will bombard the emotional part of the brain and decrease access to the memory center of the brain. This can result in "brain fog" and decreased attention span. How susceptible you are to the effects of stress on your brain has to do with your biochemical makeup.

For example, maybe you work in a high-paced, cut-throat industry and it's really taking a toll on you. You have headaches, stomach pain, and you can feel your blood pressure rising. But your coworker across the aisle, who deals with the same circumstances, seems to be faring just fine. Why are *you* the one who feels so terrible?

When you're feeling stressed, it's important to realize that it's not just the situation at hand that's making you feel lousy … it's also *your* body's unique response to the stressor. Many factors can predispose to and trigger a person's response. Previous exposure to stressors, biochemistry, genetics, environmental cues, and lifestyle patterns all affect our very individualized reactions to stressors.

Chronic exposure to stress hormones, whether it occurs during the prenatal period, infancy, childhood, adolescence, adulthood, or in aging, has an additive impact on brain structures involved in cognition and mental health. In fact, it has been demonstrated that the intensity of the stress response can depend upon interactions between your genetic makeup and prior exposure to environmental adversity, especially early in life.[32] This means that less stimulus is needed to induce a stress response if your body was already overloaded during the process of development, exposed to early-life trauma, or experienced insufficient recovery from repeated stress.[32,42]

Differing blood types are another factor contributing to the variable reactions to environmental stressors. The following comments of Dr. Ginger Nash, adapted from Dr. D'Adamo's newsletter, explains this interplay between environmental triggers and genetic predispositions:

> The gene that codes for ABO blood type ... affects other genes in close proximity that control things like dopamine metabolism, cortisol levels, and other processes that will affect the entire nervous system's coordination. For example, Type B needs additional nitrogen rich foods and supplements because their bodies lack the ability to produce a compound called nitric oxide to the extent that the other blood types do. Nitric oxide helps coordinate the nervous system, immune system and cardiovascular system.[43]

Dr. Nash goes on to say that blood types also differ in their production of cortisol, with Type A folks producing the most, and Type O's producing the least. High levels of cortisol can cause adrenal burnout, resulting in depression and fatigue in those with Type A. Type O's are more likely to respond to stress with an overproduction of adrenaline, resulting in anxiety. Over the long term, high adrenaline can also turn into depression from a burned-out nervous system.[43]

Sex Hormone Shifts

Genetics,[20,24-25] environment,[44-45] stress,[34-40] and lifestyle factors[46-47] all have an impact on our hormonal balance. Beyond any external factors, there exists the natural biological rhythm of a woman's monthly hormonal cycle. These biological fluctuations are designed to support reproduction and are vital to consider when hormonal shifts are amplified or silenced by lifestyle factors and personal choices.[47]

We talked about the effects of hormones on our biology and emotions, but how imbalances affect a premenopausal woman's overall quality-of-life and goals is also important. For example, how can a woman feel spiritually connected when she is inundated by menstrual cramps, food cravings, and a feeling of malaise? Most women will attest to how these symptoms during their menstrual cycle can impact their relationships and well-being. Many will specifically mention their mood,[10] cravings,[33] and weight. These biological imbalances can be remedied by nurturing the body back into its natural rhythm.

Normally, the body's hormonal patterns act according to the cues of this biological rhythm. For example, the ratio of estrogen to progesterone in a normal menstrual cycle regulates the process of reproduction. The rise in progesterone in the second half of the cycle helps the body to make a home for a new life; a drop in progesterone signals a shedding of the uterine lining (menstruation) when the released egg is left unfertilized. If the relationship between estrogen and progesterone is thrown off for any reason, these signals quickly become disorganized.[48]

Our toxic world contains a wide array of synthetic molecules with estrogen-like actions, called xenoestrogens. These chemicals are found in our food, personal care products, and the environment. A combination of xenoestrogens and various stressors causes many women to become "estrogen-dominant."[44-45,49] This means their estrogen activity is higher than their progesterone. This imbalance can result in menstrual issues such as heavy periods, clotting, and cramping. Estrogen dominance can be magnified by imbalanced liver function, nutrient deficiencies, and insulin resistance. As a result, PMS, cravings, mood changes, and menstrual issues can intensify.

For example, many women crave more carbohydrates close to the onset of their period. Estrogen is naturally at its highest at this time, which has an impact on serotonin receptors in the brain. This neurotransmitter not only modulates mood, digestion, and pain, but also food cravings.[50] Urges for sweets—whether due to genetic variations in serotonin receptivity,[51] blood sugar imbalances, or low stress reserve—may become even more noticeable when an estrogen-dominant pattern causes a reduction in available thyroid hormone.[13] This leaves a woman feeling fatigued and in need of a quick (processed) energy source. Unfortunately, increasing one's sugar intake only perpetuates the cycle, contributing to insulin resistance and changes in available testosterone levels. Whereas, excess testosterone and androgens in females can lead to insulin resistance and obesity;[52-54] women who have low testosterone will have a hard time maintaining lean body mass. Furthermore, those with suboptimal testosterone levels may also experience low libido,[52] which can have an impact on their significant relationships.

For these women, symptom relief can be found by implementing lifestyle behaviors and dietary patterns that help balance blood sugar, decrease stress, and modify estrogen-dominant patterns. Women should also be careful to avoid exposure to xenoestrogens (see following chapter).[44-45] Moreover, emphasizing healthy carbohydrates in the diet and providing neurotransmitter support as needed, especially during the menstrual cycle, can assist in rebalancing hormones.

Menopause

Some women go straight from PMS to menopausal nightmares. Many believe that the transition into menopause will be a turbulent rollercoaster, but this doesn't have to be the case. I've had women in my practice enter menopause without suffering any of the "typical" menopausal symptoms they expect.

The naturopathic doctor views symptoms as a means of communicating about an imbalance in the body; just as digestive issues and mood disorders indicate that something needs attention, pesky hormonal symptoms do as well. Therefore, hot flashes, mood changes, weight gain, and low libido can actually serve as guideposts for what is out of balance.

For example, as we discussed earlier in the chapter, there is a complex feedback mechanism that helps maintain proper hormone levels. The common estrogen-dominant pattern, which a woman may have experienced early in life, can be compounded by the additional stress of menopause, as well as decreased adrenal capacity to deal with it. The result can be abnormal levels of additional hormones, and soaring insulin levels. If the shifts in hormones and the stress response occur too rapidly for the brain to keep up, temperature regulation can suffer, and those dreaded sweaty hot flashes can show up. [55-56]

Key Factors for Hormonal Health

The good news is that there is a solution!

The focus should always be on finding and treating the cause. This will vary with each individual, but there are a few basic foundational treatments that will benefit most women. To begin with, the body can't properly make hormones without the appropriate raw materials obtained from a well-balanced diet.

Remember the low-fat diet craze back in the 1980s? That was not a good time for optimum health in the United States. Your body *needs* cholesterol to produce all of your sex hormones and vitamin D, as well as to make the cell membranes of every cell in your body; you also need some fat to produce cholesterol in your liver.[1,57] Eating low-fat, but consuming partially-hydrogenated fatty acids (trans fats) actually "clogs" the receptor sites of your cell membranes. This has been linked to cardiovascular disease.[58-59] Furthermore, when this happens, feedback from hormonal signals can go awry. Think of this as a major miscommunication between your gut, brain, cardiovascular, and nervous system.

It's important for your brain and body to eat the *right kinds* of fat to produce a proper balance of sex hormones and other gene expression-modulating factors, such as vitamin D. Healthy fats actually teach your body to turn on the fat-burning gene by interacting with specific receptors on fat cells.[1,57] Examples of healthy fats are omega-3 fatty acids, found in high-quality supplements and in wild-caught fish, such as salmon.

Did you know that your brain produces a hormone called brain-derived neurotrophic factor (BDNF), which can regulate hunger? Or that your fat cells make a hormone called leptin, which is responsible for signaling satiation to the brain during a meal?[60] Optimal signaling of both of these factors can be enhanced by addressing your diet.

Eating a balanced diet with whole foods, lower refined carbohydrates, and optimal levels of fat and protein can also help correct blood sugar spikes. Remember, imbalances in blood sugar can trigger surges of cortisol and insulin, which results in lower levels of estrogen and progesterone. This can explain symptoms such as mood changes, cravings, and weight gain, which I discussed in the section on estrogen-dominant patterns.

Digestive tract health is imperative in order to ensure absorption of all of the essential nutrients required to balance hormones. Because the gut is responsible for making many of our neurotransmitters (through the enteric nervous system), optimizing its function also helps correct mood imbalances. Furthermore, the colon is home to the beneficial bacteria that assist the liver in hormone detoxification.

It is wise, therefore, to support the gut with appropriate supplements as needed. Digestive enzymes can be incorporated for optimal assimilation and metabolism of nutrients. Adding probiotics and prebiotic foods can help tone down inflammation in the colon, as well as help establish an ideal home for the gut flora to thrive. Eating a diet that's rich in cruciferous vegetables (e.g., broccoli) will provide the body with the indole compound, diindolylmethane (DIM), which helps the liver reduce the amount of potent and inflammatory estrogen metabolites.[61-62] This, in turn, results in a healthier balance of estrogen and progesterone.

If a woman is experiencing intensive hormonal imbalances, herbs and essential oils that balance adrenals and other hormones can also be utilized. Herbal supplements that support estrogen balance include red clover, black cohosh, and the essential oils of sage or clary sage. Foods containing phytoestrogens and lignans, such as flax seeds and fermented soy products, can also be incorporated into the diet to optimize estrogen activity in the body.[63]

Balancing the stress response should be part of any hormonal protocol in order to prevent the stress-induced rise in cortisol that hijacks progesterone. Using adrenal tonic herbals, such as *Withania somnifera* (ashwagandha)[64] and lavender, nutmeg, and citrus essential oils, can help calm the brain and body and maximize optimal progesterone output. Nutrient support is also important and is highlighted in the next section.

The take-away point in this section is that there are many natural options available for balancing hormones. Talking to a knowledgeable integrative practitioner who will guide you in making some lifestyle and dietary changes can help you achieve an overall higher quality of life.

Hormone Replacement Therapy

Hormone replacement is a hot topic that is also quite controversial. Guidelines continue to shift as more research is revealed. Current recommendations seem to favor the lowest possible dose to treat a woman's symptoms. For many practitioners, the evidence indicating links between conventional hormone replacement and increased risk of female cancers is a concern. Risks associated with bio-identical hormonal replacement haven't been fully elucidated. Still, some evidence does suggest that bio-identical hormonal replacement, which uses biochemical equivalents of our own hormones, produces much more favorable outcomes compared to conventional hormones.[65]

I have seen how balancing lifestyle factors and providing nutritional and herbal support in the form of individualized plans relieves many women's menopausal symptoms. It may be practitioners' lack of awareness about the power of pharmaceutical-grade herbal products and the hormone regulating effects of therapeutic oils that explains why these agents aren't more commonly used. I have found it quite remarkable to learn the mechanisms of these natural products; i.e., their ability to actually upregulate or downregulate estrogen and progesterone receptor function, depending on what the body needs. (See the soy discussion in chapter 3 for more details).

One of the major factors influencing women's hormonal health, which is vital yet often ignored in conventional medicine, is the mind-body-hormonal connection.[66] As mentioned, the impact of stress on hormones is profound. Distressing thoughts can also trigger biochemical responses that produce or aggravate many symptoms.

Remember, stress impacts the adrenals, and calm adrenals means happy hormones. Thankfully, more and more research is revealing the scientific evidence behind the ancient wisdom of calming the mind for physical health. Relaxation and meditation can effectively modulate the release of stress hormones, which in turn affects the whole endocrine (hormonal) system.

One doctor in the forefront of mind-body medicine is Dr. Christiane Northrup. In her book *Women's Body, Women's Wisdom*,[67] Dr. Northrup discusses how balancing your emotional state with presence, setting boundaries on overextending yourself, proper rest, and optimal nutrition are all essential for restoring healthy adrenal gland functioning.

Here are some recommended ways to support your adrenal glands:

1. Optimal nutrition: This includes a whole-foods diet and incorporating the following adrenal-supporting nutrients as needed:
    - Vitamin D
    - Vitamin B5
    - Vitamin B12
    - Vitamin C
    - Magnesium
2. Fulfilling and supporting relationships: This will boost feel-good, stress-relieving neurotransmitters.
3. Getting proper rest: The best time to sleep for replenishing the adrenal glands is before 10 p.m. This timing is in relation to the rise and fall of cortisol levels.
4. Healthy belief patterns: Practicing positive thoughts will encourage the release of healthy hormone signals, as well as prevent the release of stress neurotransmitters.
5. A sense of purpose: This is to motivate and empower your life in order to prevent burnout from mediocrity.
6. Movement: Exercise is a potent mood-supporting tool. It also boosts circulation and aids in stress relief.
7. A safe environment: This will allow for emotional growth and optimal oxygenation to the brain.
8. Herbals or bio-identical hormones, if necessary, to help balance hormones.

Find a Happy Balance

Many women may protest, but it's true ... hormones are our friends. Our hormones are important messengers that function to keep us in balance, physically and emotionally. At the risk of repeating myself, I must reiterate that in cases of complex hormonal imbalances, it's important to have a knowledgeable practitioner measure how well your hormones are functioning. This can often be achieved through the appropriate lab tests and a detailed clinical history discussed in this chapter.

When you choose a practitioner, make sure that the he or she is trained in reading subclinical symptoms and lab values. Lab results labeled as "normal" (based on the absence of a diagnosable disease) don't necessarily mean "optimal." Your practitioner can help you establish the best protocol for rebalancing your hormones and helping you find peace of mind in a symptom-free life.

CHAPTER 8

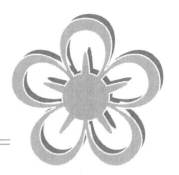

Toxic in the 21st Century

Nasty chemicals and pollutants are present in the gas we pump, the carpet and paint in our house, the apples we eat, and the water we drink. The fact is, we can't get away from our toxic environment. At least 80,000 chemicals are registered for use in the commercial industry today,[1] with about 25 percent being reported as hazardous to human health. The CDC documented the extent of pollutants in their 2009 *Fourth National Report on Human Exposure to Environmental Chemicals*[1] — a 529-page "summary" of how different aspects of environmental chemicals can harm us. The average volunteer participant in this study had over 200 chemicals in his or her blood and urine samples. Seventy-five of those documented chemicals, including acrylamide, arsenic, environmental phenols (bisphenol A and triclosan), and perchlorate, had never before been seen in humans![2]

This translates into an unprecedented level of burden being placed on the human body as it's forced to deal with toxic effects from the environment while still carrying on its normal activities. All of our organs of elimination (the liver, kidneys, lungs, colon, and skin) are especially strained under these conditions. Still, the main organ of focus, in terms of this issue, has been the liver, and for good reason ... this organ is our detoxifying powerhouse.

Furthermore, as the liver assists in removing harmful substances, it also cleanses the body of retired red blood cells, converts ammonia to urea for excretion (thereby reducing kidney burden), and breaks down hormones. Additionally, the liver is responsible for protein synthesis from amino acids, the metabolism of carbohydrates, protein, and lipids, the synthesis of platelets, blood clotting factors, angiotensinogen (a blood pressure-signaling hormone), and the formation of bile. Furthermore, your liver stores glucose, iron, copper, and vitamins A, D, and B12, and has an impact on their levels.[3]

So Why Isn't Everyone Sick?

This abundance of relatively new chemical combinations in our environment is clearly having an effect on people's health.[4-9] I see this daily in the increased number of clients who report non-specific, but very real, ailments without a known "trigger." In some sense, everyone is "sick" from man-made chemicals, even if one's symptoms may not be obviously connected to them.

Most conventional practitioners are not trained to look for symptoms of toxic burden or to recognize them, since they can be insidious. Therefore, it's common to have vague symptoms be dismissed as psychological, or to be diagnosed with a disease and treated with a medication that only addresses the effects of the environmental contributors to the disease pathology. A good example of this is the association between high blood lead levels and high blood pressure.[10] A doctor may place a patient on an anti-hypertensive drug, and over time have to increase the dosage or prescribe additional medications without ever thinking to measure levels of lead in the blood or urine. For this reason, it's wise to consider that environmental toxicity can contribute to illness by affecting how the body functions, even if it's not the sole cause of a particular disease.

Many of my clients who have limited ability to modify their environment have still experienced relief from chronic ailments when their bodies' ability to deal with these exposures was supported. This means that headaches, heart arrhythmias, skin and nail changes, muscle aches, digestive disturbances, changes in weight and appetite, fatigue, and mood imbalances can often be alleviated when the body is properly equipped to handle environmental insults.

Just as everyone responds to emotional stressors differently, not everyone is affected in the same way by environmental exposures; two people who are subject to the same pollutant can have two very different responses. One's genetic makeup,[11-12] duration and quantity of exposure, medical history, lifestyle, and other factors all influence one's reaction to toxic exposures.[10] In short, the potential of environmental illness is based on the degree of exposure to toxins over a period of time, combined with one's unique ability to remove them from the body.

> This concept is referred to as the "total toxic load" and can be expressed in the following way:
> **TOTAL TOXIC LOAD= Total Toxic Exposure minus the Ability to Mobilize, Detoxify, and Excrete Toxins**

Your unique genetic makeup can have a profound effect on this process of toxin removal and, therefore, how sensitive you are to any amount of exposure. Many disgruntled partners will attest to this fact. For example, a man may notice that his wife suffers from chronic sinusitis since the roof began leaking (mold exposure), whereas he himself may have no symptoms at all. This can lead to an unsympathetic response and sometimes even relationship issues.

Think of the relational, emotional, and physical impact of our society fully embracing the viewpoint of biochemical individuality. It would become common knowledge that just one little alteration in an enzyme's genetic sequence of DNA could make one person a powerful detoxifier, and another predisposed to diagnosis of multiple chemical sensitivity. It would enable us to view people as individuals with their unique genetic predispositions and sensitivities, versus viewing them as "unresponsive and non-compliant," or "whiney."

The good news is that genetics is only one factor in the web-like interaction of a person's entire physiological response. Digestive prowess, liver health, hormonal balance, emotional resilience, existing health conditions, medication use, nutrient reserve, and diet are just some of the major factors that will determine the likelihood of a person experiencing symptoms from environmental exposures.

For example, dairy consumption and chronic use of steroids can both negatively impact how effectively a person eliminates mold toxins from a leaky basement. A leaky lead pipe may affect an individual more profoundly if she is also experiencing digestive issues. Arsenic exposure from a playground or wood deck (or even non-organic chicken!) can affect a person with a B-vitamin deficiency more than it would affect a person taking a regular multi-vitamin that includes a good B complex.[13]

Toxic Bodies and Toxic Fat

So, now that we feel "dirty," what can we do to clean our insides?

In our modern world, cleansing the body is not only becoming increasingly necessary, but borderline trendy in the mainstream population. I have to give kudos to the prolific media coverage of cleansing, as it has shed light on the dangers of chronic environmental exposures. This marketing campaign has presented the opportunity for integrative practitioners to answer questions regarding our exposures and safe, scientific, and gentle detoxification techniques (based on the body's unique biochemistry), as opposed to the "detoxification for weight loss" fads. Long before it was popularized, naturopathic medicine has supported the notion that cleansing and detoxifying the body of "toxins" is integral to health.

Eating nutritiously is imperative if we are to equip the body to deal with all it is up against. The health status of an individual goes far beyond caloric intake and weight. If we don't have proper nourishment from the foods we eat, the liver's ability to clear out damaging environmental poisons will be diminished. Specifically, in the absence of specific nutrients, toxins that can't be cleared will accumulate in the body. This can lead to an excess of free radicals – inflammatory compounds that can cause harm to various tissues.

Too many of us think about food in terms of weight, fearful that we might become part of our nation's obesity epidemic. As a result, it's easy to compromise our health as we obsess about our looks or the numbers on a scale. For instance, you might adopt a vegan diet, not for spiritual reasons, but for weight loss. However, if your body is deprived of the key amino acids found in proteins, toxins will not be effectively bound in the liver and carried to the digestive tract for removal. This is also why fasting can cause issues for people who are nutrient-deprived, or "fat and starving to death." In this case, the body is deficient in the vital proteins needed to carry out the second phase of liver detoxification.

Without these building blocks of life, an individual who's fasting can experience vague symptoms from the toxins that float unbound through the bloodstream. Some label this response a "healing crisis" or "Herxheimer reaction"; however, this effect would be unlikely to occur if a proper cleansing technique was used that encourages binding and excretion of the problem-causing chemicals.

Furthermore, a sudden release of too many toxins into the bloodstream can cause the body to sequester and trap these offending substances in fluid or fat. Even though the body does this as a means of protection, it can result in bloated bellies, toxic fat, and difficult weight loss. If these harmful substances cannot be removed safely, the excess weight and fluid retention will remain and cause downstream negative effects on other body systems.

Fortunately, we are learning more and more about the causes and effects of environmental toxicity and the natural steps we can take to help our bodies eliminate toxins *before* they take hold and cause significant damage to our health.

What to Consider When Cleansing

Considering the hype surrounding this topic, I realize that some folks will want to try cleansing on their own. The concern I have with most commercially available detoxification protocols is that they typically don't take into account your own unique biochemistry, health status, detoxification capacity, and your total toxic load of environmental exposures. Moreover, the most important point to remember, when undertaking any detoxification or cleansing program, is to make sure that your bowels are able to effectively clear out the toxic byproducts released from your liver and kidneys. Unfortunately, many over-the-counter detoxification products only work to stimulate the liver, which means that all those toxins from the liver can now more easily accumulate in your bloodstream.

So, although there are many "detoxing" and "cleansing" products on the market today, I would caution you to forego doing it alone, and encourage you instead to find a healthcare practitioner who can implement all of the above detoxification considerations for you. I have found this individualized approach to detoxification to work well for my clients. In fact, some marvel at how easy it is when they don't have to worry about "detox reactions" – a result of being supplied with everything the body needs to rid itself of toxins.

Below are tips for you to consider if you plan on cleansing. These will help to ensure that your body will be supported rather than stressed during the process:

1. Avoid water and juice fasts if you don't have medical supervision. These types of fasts mobilize toxins without supplying your body with the nutrients it needs to remove them effectively. This can lead to harmful side effects and potential damage to the body. Furthermore, our world is much more toxic today than when these techniques were first implemented, resulting in an even greater mobilization of harmful substances. Being monitored for safety is critical.
2. Make sure you are on high-quality nutrients. For example, your body needs the B vitamins and minerals that assist enzymes in the liver to convert toxins to harmless compounds that can then be excreted from the body. This conversion occurs in phases of biotransformation. In phase I, the liver prepares the toxins for the next phase; in phase II, these compounds are bound and made more water-soluble, so that they can be safely eliminated. Without having adequate nutrients on board, the toxins can get stuck in one of these phases, and recirculate into the body.
3. Gut integrity is a must. Harmful compounds must be moved out of the liver and into the colon (and kidneys) for removal. This is why I devoted a whole chapter to our "inner tube" … the gut plays a role in everything! So, make sure to give your intestines first priority by optimizing their functioning before starting any liver or kidney cleanse!
4. Protect your body from the inflammation produced during toxin biotransformation. For example, if these chemicals get stuck in Phase 1, the associated free radical production can cause tissue damage. Therefore, adding antioxidants and fish oil to a cleansing protocol can provide needed protection and ensure

a more comfortable cleanse. Some good antioxidant examples are CoQ10, essential oils, krill oil (a type of plankton that contains both essential fatty acids and the antioxidant astaxanthin), selenium, vitamin C, and molybdenum.

5. Make sure you have enough protein. Consider using whey-based or pea-based amino acid protein supplements, to give your body the amino acids it needs to carry out Phase 2 detoxification and also prevent muscle breakdown from weight loss. I usually advise against rice protein, as 2010 and 2012 analyses by Consumer Reports indicated it can be contaminated with metals and its high-carbohydrate content can cause blood sugar issues in some people.

6. Make sure you sweat, to effectively recycle toxins from the blood into the lymph. Your sweat glands release toxins that other organs of excretion can't! If you're unable to sweat, you may be more toxic, and if you don't move and sweat, you aren't mobilizing toxins for removal.

    (A note of caution: Using a sauna to mobilize toxins without first ensuring proper excretory function and nutritional support can result in severe side effects; thus, sweat the natural way – through exercise – if you aren't being monitored.)

7. Water, water, water! Hydrating with plenty of water is crucial for various bodily functions, especially elimination of toxins.

The Importance of Clean Eating in a Dirty World

If you've followed these recommendations that support your body during a cleanse, make sure you're not introducing additional pesticides and chemicals into your body through your diet. We can't control the environment, but we *can* control our toxic exposure through our dietary choices. Don't think of your meals as bundles of calories, think of them as potentially powerful cleansing agents containing information that will guide the body to health. We can still eat yummy, nutritious foods that provide the potent phytochemicals that help our detoxification systems remove pesticides, herbicides, and other toxins, and also help heal the body from their toxic effects.

A big obstacle to making this choice simple is the mass marketing that encourages us to ignore food quality and focus instead on eating for pleasure. We are lured into spending money on nutrient-depleted foods containing addictive substances, rather than investing in foods that will heal our bodies and keep them healthy. Ronnie Cummins from the Organic Consumers Association asks some very eye-opening questions on this topic:

> *Did you ever vote to allow corporate agribusiness to spray a billion pounds of toxic pesticides, and dump 24 billion pounds of climate-destabilizing chemical fertilizers on U.S. crops and farmlands every year? Did you give the OK for factory farms, so-called Confined Animal Feeding Operations (CAFOs), to feed billions of hapless creatures massive amounts of genetically engineered grain, antibiotics, hormones, steroids, blood, manure, and slaughterhouse waste? Did you give Monsanto, Dow, and Dupont permission to "modify" so-called "conventional" supermarket, school cafeteria, and restaurant food with genetically engineered bacteria, viruses, foreign DNA, and antibiotic-resistant genes?*[14]

Most folks are not aware that our foods are altered in these ways. Even when we think we're making healthy choices, we may not be. For example, that apple we're reaching for may be contaminated with pesticides or is genetically modified. However, now that you're aware of these dangers, it's important to be responsible and proactive with this information. By choosing high-quality, organic, non-processed foods and eating a whole foods diet, we can lessen the total toxic load and stress on our biotransformation process.

Tips for Making Our Bodies Safe in a Scary World

After following tips for safe cleansing, some other everyday support measures can help ensure that your liver doesn't get overloaded again! For example, it may be helpful to incorporate protective nutrients into your daily self-care regimen, including specific antioxidants (such as CoQ10), fiber, probiotics, and nutrients such as vitamins C, E, B, magnesium, and selenium.

Prevention is the best medicine! Here are some additional general recommendations that can prevent toxic overload and keep you healthy in this chemical-laden world:

1. Eat organic foods whenever possible. As mentioned, organic foods are not only more nutritious, but also less toxic.
2. Use a filtered water system to reduce your exposure to substances that can harm the body, such as fluoride, chlorine, lead, and various bacteria, parasites, and pathogens.
3. Consider using diindolylmethane (DIM). This compound can help the liver detoxify inflammatory estrogen compounds that derive from either your own cellular metabolism or from the environment. DIM is available in supplement form, but is also found in cruciferous vegetables, such as broccoli and Brussels sprouts. Crucifers can also protect us from toxicity from lead and other toxins, since they contain glucoraphanin. This compound is the precursor to sulforaphane, which modulates liver enzymes that assist in the safe removal and excretion of toxins.[15]
4. Control your gut bugs! Consume a good source of probiotics in a supplement or in healthy fermented foods. These little critters in your gastrointestinal tract help prevent enterohepatic recycling of toxins (recirculation of toxins back to the liver and into the bloodstream), thereby enhancing your cleansing capability. Also, remember to feed them healthy fiber!

There are some cautions regarding probiotic use, however. For example, if you have excess yeast or small bowel bacterial overgrowth, probiotics can create some serious gas issues. Be sure to check with your healthcare provider if you are experiencing these symptoms.[16] Furthermore, if gastrointestinal yeast overgrowth is an issue, natural or prescription antifungals may be needed before using probiotics or any other intervention. This is in order to first calm down the immune system by clearing out any infection and its production of toxic byproducts.

5. Eat chocolate! Well, this recommendation specifically pertains to eating high-quality, raw cocoa found in dark chocolate. It can be a pleasurable way to provide the body with flavonoids – antioxidants that support microcirculation. A word of caution is necessary here: chocolate can have the "good" processed out by added sugar, milk, and hydrogenation. Therefore, look for dark chocolate made from raw, organic cocoa, to obtain these powerful molecules.

These flavonoids will "speak" to your genes, helping them to function more effectively, and provide health benefits such as boosting your intestinal health and immunity. Cocoa has also been shown to decrease the risk of cardiometabolic disorders, and to lower blood pressure, calm inflammation, modulate insulin resistance, and assist with vascular function.[17,18]

So, swap that average Hershey bar, filled with gooey filled caramel and white chocolate chips, for organic, raw, dark chocolate (ideally at 72 percent or higher cocoa), to receive all the benefits mentioned above.

6. Diffuse therapeutic essential oils. They can help neutralize and kill airborne toxins. At the same time, they will support your brain function and boost your health (see Chapter 6 for more details).

7. Dying to be beautiful? When choosing cosmetics and cleansers, select only personal care and household items that are chemical-free and organic. Remember, your skin is the largest organ in your body – what you put on it is absorbed and processed by the liver. For example, studies have shown that prior to leaving the house each day, the average woman exposes herself to over 168 chemicals, between her makeup, hair products, and other personal care items.[19] A nursing mother releases 20 percent of her toxic load into the baby. Why increase the burden on our poor, overly-stressed livers with toxic hair spray, when we can use natural gels and sprays?

8. Spice up and shed pounds. Spices help with weight control in a few different ways. For instance, they help to control inflammation and regulate blood sugar balance. A recent article in the *European Journal of Nutrition* highlighted the nutrigenomic properties of the spice curcumin. The researchers found that this Indian spice can reduce the risk of insulin resistance and other obesity-related conditions, such as hyperglycemia (high blood sugar) and hyperlipidemia (lipid abnormalities in the blood).[20]

    Another example of support from Mother Nature is the sweet spice, cinnamon. It has also been shown to help modulate healthy lipids and assist with blood sugar management.[21-23] Furthermore, cinnamon's antioxidant properties[11] may enable it to reduce stress on the body as it cleanses. So, sprinkle cinnamon in your tea, on your gluten-free oatmeal, or on any other healthy food for further weight-optimizing support.

9. Tea time! A recent study showed that the compound epigallocatechin gallate (EGCG), found in green tea, aids in balancing cholesterol.[24] For those who enjoy a variety of teas, oolong also contains protective antioxidants, including EGCG,

which may also calm excess inflammation and balance blood sugar.[13]

10. Subdue inflammation by applying essential oils. Inflammation encourages the accumulation of toxins, promotes tissue damage, and makes the body hold onto excess pounds. Frankincense (from the herb *Boswellia*) has been known for ability to modulate inflammation for quite some time.[26] There are different species of *Boswellia* with different properties. For example, *Boswellia sacra* has a higher content of the constituent alpha pinene, which can be used for fungal and microbial infections, compared to *Boswellia carteri*.[27]

Although both forms are therapeutic, the selection of species should be based on your main goal. For example, if you have a Candida infection that's contributing to inflammation and difficulty in losing weight, the antifungal mechanism of alpha-pinene in *Boswellia sacra* may be your best choice. In one vitro study, alpha-pinene played a significant role in inhibiting and killing *Candida albicans*.[27] In oil form, this herb can be a powerful part of a cleansing program (under the supervision of a healthcare provider), in the case of mold and yeast exposure.

Finally, targeted antioxidants are useful for individuals who are genetically predisposed to problems with detoxification. These nutrients can be given in large, therapeutic doses in such cases, and are best provided by your healthcare practitioner.

Dirty Energy

An overlooked environmental factor that may be negatively impacting our biochemistry is electromagnetic frequencies (EMFs), cell phones being a major source. Recently, the International Agency for Research on Cancer (IARC) issued a warning on the dangers of this exposure:

"After reviewing all the evidence available, the IARC working group classified radiofrequency electromagnetic fields as possibly carcinogenic to humans," panel chairman Jonathan Samet, MD, chair of preventive medicine at the USC Keck School of Medicine, said at a news teleconference. "We reached this conclusion based on a review of human evidence showing increased risk of glioma, a malignant type of brain cancer, in association with wireless phone use."[28]

Electrical devices may also affect our physiology by disrupting our circadian rhythms. A rodent study[29] found that the abnormal wake and sleep cycles resulting from EMF exposure affected not only brain health, but affected weight, metabolism, and emotions:

> *Housing in these conditions results in accelerated weight gain and obesity, as well as changes in metabolic hormones. In the brain, circadian-disrupted mice exhibit a loss of dendritic length and decreased complexity of neurons in the prelimbic prefrontal cortex, a brain region important in executive function and emotional control. Disrupted animals show decreases in cognitive flexibility and changes in emotionality consistent with the changes seen in neural architecture.*[29]

This study demonstrated how environmentally-produced disruptions in circadian rhythms impact the brain and body of animals. The findings could easily translate to humans in their own living and working conditions.

To prevent these effects and protect your brain, it would be wise to turn off your computer or cell phone, at least for a little while each day. There is added benefit in doing this: according to a study in the *Journal of Epidemiology and Community Health*, people who participate in real-life connection experiences have an overall greater satisfaction with life.[30]

Aside from taking an "information vacation" by powering off our devices, the impact of environmental EMFs can be mitigated with some of these simple tips:

1. Text instead of talk, or use a speaker phone.
2. Use a direct connection instead of Wi-Fi, whenever possible.
3. Turn off Wi-Fi routers at night, which will help your body enter the natural rhythm of sleep.
4. Switch your cell phone to "airplane mode" whenever it's near your body, and do not store the phone in your clothes.
5. Limit the hours that children use their phones, due to their heightened susceptibility.

Emotional Toxicity

It's not only our environment that can make us ill and "toxic." The ways in which we emotionally respond to stress, relationships, responsibilities, and disappointments all have an effect on our health as well. We are one of the only societies in which mind and body are deemed separate entities, yet the two are intimately connected. For example, stress and grief can cause changes in neurotransmitter signaling. As a result, hormonal, digestive, immune, and many other biochemical responses are altered. This resultant physical stress can further impact our mood and make us feel worn down.

This means it's important to stop and listen to our bodies and to be aware of what's happening emotionally when we are in certain social situations. By understanding our reactions and how they affect us physically, we will be more inclined to make different choices and respond more favorably the next time we are in a similar situation. This will result in a more stabilized and optimized biochemical response. After all, the results of any cleansing program only last so long if we are stuck in unhealthy, stressful patterns. Although it may be hard to break our familiar and patterned reactions to drama, or "comfortable discomfort," this kind of mental strain sets off inflammatory molecules and depletes vital nutrient reserves.

Consequently, it's essential to cleanse the mind, not just the body, to ensure optimal health. Below are some ideas that you can begin implementing into your life now:

1. Take time-outs from stress each day. Today it's easy to find an online course or YouTube video on relaxation or meditation to assist you with this. Practicing these techniques will help break negative brain feedback patterns and foster healthier emotional responses. By placing value on down-time, you can craft a sacred and rejuvenating space that facilitates better body and brain resilience.
2. Nurture your relationships with loved ones. Supportive and loving friendships boost feel-good brain chemicals like oxytocin and dopamine. This will reduce stress while positively impacting the immune system.
3. Try to decrease the amount of time spent with computers, news, and gadgets. Information overload can cause our bodies to be on constant "alert," and can actually increase inflammation in the body! By taking time for respite from your chronic busyness, and enjoying the present moment, your stress will diminish. Many spiritual gurus tout "success," not as a destination that necessitates compromise of joy and fulfillment, but rather a measure of how well you simply enjoy your life and what is already present in front of you.
4. Find nurturing foods that are also pleasurable to you. For example, consider a sliver of dark chocolate for a healthy treat. A study in the *Journal of Proteome Research* concluded that 40 grams of dark chocolate over a two-week period increased the removal of stress hormones from the body.[31]

Putting It All Together: Holistic and Comprehensive Support for Cleansing and Toxicity

Unfortunately, we can't escape the fact that we are surrounded by toxic chemicals, pollutants, and other foreign substances every single day of our lives. Compound this fact by the current levels of stress in the general population, and these chemicals have the potential to wreak even more serious havoc, since stress downregulates our body's ability to cleanse itself of them.

The goal should be to first rid the body of toxic burdens that are affecting health, and then to prevent future buildup of these toxins that can cause disease. As mentioned, this is a big topic in naturopathic and functional medicine because biotransformation in the liver doesn't just affect detoxification of chemicals; it also assists in most other functions, including hormonal balance, inflammation, cholesterol formation, and fat and vitamin absorption.

Some of us may feel overwhelmed when learning this information, but it would be counter productive to stress-out, feel victimized, or become hyper-diligent and seclude oneself inside a plastic bubble. The purpose of providing you with this information is to empower you with knowledge about how to supply the body with what it needs to eliminate toxins and live a more vital, healthier life.

Healthy Detoxing in a Partnership of Support

For a truly complete and optimal physical cleanse, I highly recommend working with a natural health practitioner. It's not that the process is insurmountably difficult; it's that you'll experience much better results when you spend your time, efforts, and resources on a program that's been built specifically to address *your* unique body's needs. You just can't find such a program on the shelf at a natural foods or supplement store.

Also, remember that nurturing the mind-body balance is part of complete health. If you detox your body without clearing your mind of nagging or negative thoughts, you will have accomplished only half the job. Make the commitment to a *total* detoxification of your life. A truly integrative practitioner can be your cheerleader for positive change.

CHAPTER 9

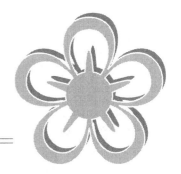

Heart & Soul Medicine

So far, we've discussed multiple major organ systems and how to keep them balanced, cleansed, and optimally healthy. However, we have not looked at what could possibly be the most important system. Its four-chambered pumping organ is responsible for delivering all of those amazing nutrients into the fully integrated body that you've achieved through the previous chapters. Our cardiovascular system is set up to do this in pretty remarkable ways – there is a lot of power in this small centralized organ!

According to the Cleveland Clinic,[1]

- Your blood vessels, consisting of arteries, veins, and capillaries, are over 60,000 miles long.
- The adult heart pumps approximately 2,000 gallons of blood through the body each day.
- Your heart beats about 100,000 times per day and will beat more than 2.5 trillion times over 70 years.
- A women's heart weighs about 8 ounces, and a man's heart weighs about 10 ounces. It is about the size of two fists.

This is why I've "saved the best for last" – it's important that we're delivering optimal nutrition and oxygen to all of our organs, not more effectively pumping more toxins and inflammatory mediators through our circulation! The heart is very active and needs optimized nutrition for its health, as well as its support of whole-body health.

Unfortunately, our nation's overall heart health is in danger. The health management initiative, "Healthy You," had this to say about the need for The American Heart Association's American Heart Month:

> *American Heart Month is a time to battle cardiovascular disease and educate Americans on what we can do to live heart-healthy lives. Heart disease, including stroke, is the leading cause of death for men and women in the United States, killing an estimated 630,000 Americans each year. It's the leading cause of death for both men and women.*
>
> *You are at higher risk of heart disease if you are:*
> - *A woman age 55 or older*
> - *A man age 45 or older*
> - *A person with a family history of early heart disease*[2]

The good news is heart disease risk factors can be mitigated by several lifestyle practices, including...

- maintaining a healthy weight
- not smoking
- maintaining healthy blood lipid levels
- avoiding alcohol
- eating a healthy diet and exercising
- managing stress

These heart-healthy lifestyle shifts are empowering ways to change any chronic disease pattern. Nonetheless, I find the above guidelines lacking in two ways:

1. They don't give the complete picture of what is important for overall heart health and ignore key risk factors. For example, did you know that oxidative stress, inflammation, infections, emotions, and lack of social support can all increase your risk of heart disease? This is why addressing these issues is vital not just for the reasons mentioned in the previous chapters, but for cardiovascular health as well.
2. Preventative medicine at its best should be based on the individual and his or her own unique needs. It is not simply about following generalized recommendations, avoiding damaging behaviors, or pharmaceutically correcting a symptom that might have resulted from not implementing these suggestions to begin with.

However, many people with heart disease attempt to make up for unhealthy and non-nourishing lifestyle choices by taking a pill or supplement. This doesn't work, for two major reasons:

1. As mentioned, conventional medicine guidelines for using pharmaceuticals to treat the heart are not aimed at treating the cause, but rather at suppressing the symptoms. This may be helpful – and even necessary – in the short term, but in the long term can cause more problems if the underlying issues aren't addressed.
2. The diseases of the heart are more than physical – we should no longer ignore the mind-spirit connection.

The Flaws in Treating Every Heart Ill with a Pill

It's not that medications aren't sometimes necessary. They're needed at times to prevent a potentially fatal outcome; however, they can also obscure the warning signs of an unhealthy heart by masking inflammatory or stress symptoms. Furthermore, using a drug to control symptoms can often lead to side effects, then additional drugs to control these side effects, and eventually the creation of a poly-pharmacy of drugs and supplements. In the end, it is hard to distinguish a bodily symptom from an "adverse drug response," and the consumer can be left feeling victimized and powerless. These are not heart-enhancing emotions!

For example, let's look at a debated topic between integrative and conventional medicine, that being cholesterol. Medical experts proclaim that taking medications to suppress the liver's manufacturing of this critical steroid is an important way to prevent cardiovascular disease. The problem with this viewpoint is that cholesterol is actually an important compound with numerous health benefits, including its role in brain support and the formation of steroid hormones and vitamin D. Moreover, it can help protect the heart from damage by controlling oxidative stress.

From a common sense point of view, think of the implications of taking a medicine that stops the formation of a compound used by every cell of the body and to make vitamin D. Besides the potential side effects of this biochemical manipulation, studies have not convincingly proven the benefits of suppressing cholesterol in most cases, and tend to be skewed to report favorable results.[3-8] Wouldn't it make more sense to address the *underlying cause* of why your body is making extra cholesterol to begin with? Furthermore, taking into account gender, age, and medical history of the population given these medications might well prevent unnecessary adverse effects.[3-10]

A good example of individualizing treatment can be found in the way heart disease expresses itself in men versus women. This gender difference is often not taken into account, in terms of dosage recommendations for medications and supplements. For example, most trials use male subjects. This fact ignores the unique hormonal modifications of cholesterol in women. Therefore, the recommendation to take a medication according to a one-size-fits-all medical theory may be overlooking the biochemical uniqueness of half of our population.[9,10]

Beyond Numbers for Heart Health

When the body is balanced and the heart is healthy, it responds in a way that keeps us strong. The heart has its own "brain," promoting healing effects through the production of specific heart hormones. Furthermore, our thoughts can trigger either helpful or harmful chemicals that are released into our circulation. Resulting feedback to our heart perpetuates the recycling of these signaling molecules.

Beyond the physical needs of the heart, there is an even more important factor for optimal cardiovascular function. The heart needs to 'feel' a sense of connection. Beyond numbers and weight, if we feel a sense of isolation, the effect of that on the physical heart is strain. In fact, social isolation, alone, has been found to be an independent predictor of death from coronary heart disease![11]

So, it isn't just a cliché – emotions do play a big part in heart health. In fact, studies exist today that prove that a heart attack can be caused by a "broken heart." According to an article in the journal, *Circulation*,

> *Acute psychological stress is associated with an abrupt increase in the risk of cardiovascular events ... [Among the 1.985 subjects], the incidence rate of acute MI [myocardial infarction] onset was elevated 21.1-fold ... within 24 hours*

of the death of a significant person and declined steadily on each subsequent day.[12]

Commenting on this study, Dr. Mercola offered additional insight regarding this link between grief and heart health in one of his articles.[13] He feels that the mechanism probably relates to levels of stress hormones in the body:

> The study did not get into the causes of the abrupt increase in risk of cardiovascular events like heart attack, but it's likely related to the flood of stress hormones your body is exposed to following extreme stress.
>
> For instance, adrenaline increases your blood pressure and your heart rate, and it's been suggested it may lead to narrowing of the arteries that supply blood to your heart, or even bind directly to heart cells allowing large amounts of calcium to enter and render the cells temporarily unable to function properly.
>
> Interestingly, while your risk of heart attack increases following severe stress, so does your risk of what's known as stress cardiomyopathy — or "broken heart syndrome" — which is basically a "temporary" heart attack that occurs due to stress.[13]

Emotional Heart Health

As discussed, heart-healthy tips go way beyond a statin prescription and medicine based on the "numbers." As an example, the American Heart Association recently recommended this integration of mind and body through the practice of yoga.[14] This is accomplished not only by yoga's effect on stress management and emotional state, but also by its powerful physical benefits:

> *Thinking prevention? As part of an overall healthy lifestyle, Cunningham said yoga can help lower blood pressure, increase lung capacity, and improve respiratory function and heart rate, and boost circulation and muscle tone. It can also improve your overall well-being while offering strength-building benefits.*
>
> *Yoga also has proven benefits for those who have faced cardiac arrest, heart attack or other heart event, according to Cunningham.*[14]

The bottom line is that for any organ system, we need to integrate change on more than just a symptom-suppressing, disease-fighting level. Naturopathic and functional medicine provide the missing piece in accomplishing this because they partner with the patient and treat the individual.

CHAPTER 10

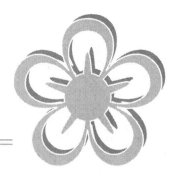

Conclusion

Moving Forward with This Book

Congratulations! If you've reached the end of this book, you're now empowered with knowledge to BreakFree from victimhood in disease-management and to become truly healthy. The next step is up to you. Only you can implement the changes that can get you to where you want to be, living your life with more joy and vitality.

Now that you have an understanding of why you are doing things in certain ways, I suggest going back to the tips listed in each chapter, starting with Chapter 1. This can be a fast or slow process, depending on your personality and how you learn most effectively.

For instance, when making the dietary changes described in the digestion section, you can either do a complete overhaul straightaway, or go a slower pace. A slower version might consist of one or two weeks of replacing your breakfast with a gluten-free option and increased protein content. After that, you could follow up with the same scenario for lunch during Weeks 3 and 4. Soon, your whole diet will be full of anti-inflammatory, nourishing foods!

Still, I wouldn't try to change everything all at once because it's easy to get overwhelmed and give up. It's generally a gradual process to retrain the brain and heart neural pathways (cybernetic set points) that have been built over time. Mind-body medicine, essential oils, and nutrients will help to support positive shifts in beliefs, which will guide you to optimally care for your body, versus giving into cravings and unhealthy patterns.

The take home message is this: Supply your body with nutrients, movement, and healthy food choices that work with your genetics, unique biochemistry, and emotional health, and it will hum for you! Using the suggestions in this book *will* help you to rebalance and reclaim your health!

We can revolutionize our healthcare system, not by changing insurance, but by changing how we think about our health, one person at a time.

EPILOGUE

EMPOWERING YOURSELF TO STAY HEALTHY

In today's society, we don't place enough value on our wellness. We are trained away from investing in our bodies, beyond superficial treatments for skin, nails, and hair. The result is that medical decisions are based on co-payments for managed care and generalized medical protocols rather than on achieving wellness according to what's best for each individual. If our current choices were making our nation healthier, slimmer, and increasing our longevity, I wouldn't be writing this book. However, we aren't that lucky. Instead, we are getting fatter and sicker, and infant mortality rates continue to rise!

Many of us are still hoping that someone will discover that powerful, almighty panacea, the fountain of youth in a pill that promises to keep us healthy, strong, and youthful while still continuing our hyperactive pace, destructive lifestyles, and poor eating habits. This is neither realistic nor self-nurturing.

America *is* growing sicker, not just physically, but in a deeply-entrenched, soul-sickness kind of way. We are taught that we deserve a break by numbing ourselves with entertainment and sugary desserts, rather than by treating ourselves to true relaxation, nourishing foods, and time to recharge with loved ones.

I wrote *BreakFree Medicine* as a means of empowering our society to truly heal from the inside out, and to break away from the mind-numbing tactics of the media. It is not inevitable that age comes with being decrepit.

I want you to truly be well ... not just for a longer life with fewer symptoms, but also in a healthier, happier, cleaner world where you are vital, strong, and able to participate in your life in ways that maximize your soul's purpose. May you and your loved ones come to know the experience of living a soul-filled and harmonious life, now and always.

ABOUT THE AUTHOR

Sarah LoBisco, ND, is a graduate of the University of Bridgeport's College of Naturopathic Medicine (UBCNM). She is licensed in Vermont as a naturopathic doctor and holds a Bachelor of Psychology from State University of New York at Geneseo. Dr. LoBisco speaks professionally on integrative medical topics, has several journal publications, and is a candidate for postdoctoral certification in functional medicine. Dr. LoBisco currently incorporates her training in holistic medical practices and conventional medicine through writing, researching, private practice, and through her independent contracting work for companies regarding supplements, nutraceuticals, essential oils, and medical foods. Dr. LoBisco also enjoys continuing to educate and empower her readers through her blogs and social media. Her recent blogs about living naturally in our complex world and on the applications of essential oils can be found at www.dr-lobisco.com and at www.saratoga.com/living-well.

GLOSSARY

Acetylcholine: A major neurotransmitter that functions to calm the central nervous system and assist with muscle contraction.

Adiponectin: A protein hormone involved in multiple metabolic functions. It is particularly helpful in protecting against type 2 diabetes. Adinopectin is produced by adipose (fat) tissue.

Adrenals: Glands that are located above the kidneys and are responsible for secreting the stress hormone cortisol and the neurotransmitters epinephrine and norepinephrine. The adrenal glands also regulate electrolytes and fluid balance via the hormone aldosterone.

Body mass index (BMI): A measurement that estimates the amount of fat in a person's body. It is calculated based on one's weight and height.

Celiac disease: An autoimmune disorder in which an immune reaction to the gliadin protein found in gluten promotes inflammation in the small intestine.

Cholecystokinin: A digestive hormone in the small intestine responsible for metabolizing fat and protein.

Circadian rhythm: The body's internal clock that controls the patterns of sleep, wakefulness, and hunger that occur regularly over a 24-hour period.

Cortisol: A hormone released by the adrenal glands. Cortisol ultimately raises blood sugar in response to stress or low blood sugar levels, and is also responsible for suppressing the inflammatory response.

Cybernetic set point: The baseline "normal" for a controlled system; for the purposes of our discussion, the system is the human body.

Demulcent herbs: Herbs that have soothing effects on mucous membranes, such as in the respiratory and gastrointestinal tracts.

Epigenetics: The study of changes in gene expression due to environmental factors.

Estrogen-dominant pattern: A condition in which estrogen activity in the body is not sufficiently balanced with progesterone. This imbalance can cause premenstrual and menstrual symptoms.

GABA (gamma-aminobutyric acid): The chief inhibitory neurotransmitter in the brain. Its principal role is to decrease excitability in the nervous system and to control muscle tone and heart rate.

Genotype: The specific genetic makeup of a person, usually as it relates to a specific gene.

Genotropic theory: A theory based on the concept that the aging process is linked to genetic changes.

Genotropism: A theory that concludes that instinct is biological and genetic in origin.

Glucose: A sugar produced by the body as an important source of energy.

Glutamate: A neurotransmitter that plays an important role in learning and memory. It tends to be excitatory but is sometimes inhibitory; it is also the precursor to GABA.

Gluten: A protein found in many wheat and grain products. It can cause a wide array of symptoms in people who are susceptible to celiac disease and/or gluten sensitivity.

Hormesis: A concept in toxicology based on low-dose stimulation and high-dose inhibition. In medicine, it is a method of finding the correct dosage based on the dose response curve that shows the greatest effect at the lowest dose. An increase in this dose can have a negative effect or no effect.

Hypoglycemia: A low level of glucose in the bloodstream. Cortisol is usually released to correct the imbalance.

Hyperglycemia: A high level of glucose in the bloodstream. Insulin is typically released to correct the imbalance.

Insulin: A hormone produced by the pancreas. Insulin moves glucose into the cells, to be used for energy.

Insulin resistance: A condition in which the insulin produced by the pancreas becomes less effective at lowering blood sugar levels. As a result, blood sugar levels can remain high and contribute to various health problems, including type 2 diabetes and heart disease.

Intestinal permeability: A condition in which the wall of the intestine becomes too permeable between cells, allowing bacterial toxins and undigested food particles to enter the system. It is also called "leaky gut."

Leaky gut: Excess permeability of the intestine that allows toxins and small molecules to escape into the body.

Leptin: A hormone produced by fat cells that is responsible for decreasing appetite. If leptin levels are low or the body is resistant to its signal, satiety is not achieved. This can lead to overeating and obesity.

Malabsorption: A condition in which food and nutrients are not properly absorbed from the small intestine. It can lead to malnutrition and issues related to nutritional deficiencies.

Microflora: A collective name given to the bacteria and other microorganisms that normally reside in the gastrointestinal tract.

Neurotransmitter: A chemical agent that is responsible for transmitting signals in the nervous system. Many neurotransmitters are synthesized by the gut's own nervous system, called the enteric nervous system.

Orthorexia: A pathological obsession with being healthy, in which a person develops an extreme aversion to foods considered to be unhealthy.

Panacea: A (non-existent) cure for all ailments.

Probiotics: Live microorganisms found in supplements, yogurt, fermented foods, and some yeasts. They generally have important health benefits.

Phenotype: The observable traits and behaviors that result from the interaction between environmental influences and a person's genetic makeup and gene expression.

Phytonutrients: Natural constituents of plants that are believed to have healthful benefits for the human body.

Serotonin: A neurotransmitter found in the gastrointestinal tract, as well as the central nervous system and platelets. Serotonin is believed to be largely responsible for feelings of contentment and happiness.

Sesquiterpenes: Natural compounds present in some essential oils which stimulate the glands; they have anti-inflammatory properties, can cross the blood-brain barrier, and also help the body to function optimally.

Trans fats: Fat that has been chemically modified by hydrogenation to improve shelf life. Trans fats are not recognized by the body, and can significantly contribute to heart disease and other illnesses.

Total toxic load: The result of a person's toxic exposures over a period of time, compounded by their own unique ability to remove toxins from the body.

WGA: Wheat germ agglutinin, a protein found in gluten that is thought to contribute to the negative effects of gluten ingestion.

Resources: for Further Reading

Read my blogs about living naturally in our complex world at http://www.dr-lobisco.com/, and also at http://www.saratoga.com/living-well/sarah-lobisco.html.

To learn more about integrative and natural approaches to health and wellness, explore these sites, or other works by these authors:

American Association of Naturopathic Medicine: www.naturopathic.org

Institute for Functional Medicine: www.functionalmedicine.org

Green Med Info: www.greenmedinfo.com

Dr. Mark Hyman: www.drhyman.com

Dr. Christiane Northrup: www.drnorthrup.com

Dr. Daniel Amen: www.amenclinics.com

Dr. Joseph Mercola: www.mercola.com

Hayhouse Radio. www.hayhouseradio.com

REFERENCES BY CHAPTER

Chapter 1

1. Null G, Dean C, Feldman M, et al. *Death by Medicine*. Edinburg, VA: Axios Press; 2011. Available at http://www.whale.to/a/null9.html. Accessed February 23, 2012.
2. James JT. A new, evidence-based estimate of patient harms associated with hospital care. *J Patient Saf.* 2013;9(3):122-128. Available at: http://www.trustfor.com/uploads/1/6/3/0/16302268/a new evidence based estimate of patient harms.2.pdf. Accessed June 13, 2014.
3. Davis K, Schoen C, Stremikis K. Mirror, Mirror on the Wall: How the Performance of the U.S. Health Care System Compares Internationally, 2010 Update. June 23, 2010. The Commonwealth Fund Web site. http://www.commonwealthfund.org/Publications/Fund-Reports/2010/Jun/Mirror-Mirror-Update.aspx?page=all. Accessed February 23, 2012.
4. Landrigan CP, Parry GJ, Bones CB, et al. Temporal trends in rates of patient harm resulting from medical care. *N Engl J Med.* 2010;363(22):2124-2134.
5. Budnitz DS, Pollock DA, Weidenbach KN, et al. National surveillance of emergency department visits for outpatient adverse drug events. *JAMA.* 2006;296(15):1858-1866.
6. Rubio M, Bousquet PB, Demoly P. Update in drug allergy: novel drugs with novel reaction patterns. *Curr Opin Allergy Clin Immunol.* 2010;10(5):457-462. Available at: http://www.medscape.com/viewarticle/730658 1. Accessed February 23, 2012.
7. American Medical Association. The Medicare Physician Payment Schedule. AMA Web site. http://www.ama-assn.org/ama/pub/physician-resources/solutions-managing-your-practice/coding-billing-insurance/medicare/the-medicare-physician-payment-schedule.shtml. Accessed February 23, 2012.

8. Kirsch M. Is physician decision-making as ethical as we think? November, 1999. *ACP Internist* Web site. http://www.acpinternist.org/archives/1999/11/ethical.htm. Accessed February 23, 2012.
9. Dawkins R. Is Science a Religion? Skeptical Science Web site. http://www.skeptical-science.com/essays/science-religion-richard-dawkins/. First published in the *Humanist*, January/February, 1997. Accessed February 23, 2012.
10. The Pros and Cons of Evidence-based Medicine as It Relates to the Practice of Natural Medicine. Clinical Roundtable (Audio). Tina Kaczor talks with Richard Barrett, ND and Andrew Shao, PhD. *Natural Medicine Journal*. November, 2010.
11. Melander H, Ahlqvist-Rastad J, Meijer MG, Beermann B. Evidence b(i)ased medicine—selective reporting from studies sponsored by pharmaceutical industry: review of studies in new drug applications. *BMJ*. 2003;326:1171. Available at: http://www.bmj.com/content/326/7400/1171. Accessed February 23, 2012.
12. Ullman D. How Scientific is Modern Medicine Really? *Huffington Post*. June 20, 2010. Available at: http://www.huffingtonpost.com/dana-ullman/how-scientific-is-modern b 543158.html. Accessed February 23, 2012.
13. Rosenbloom M. Vitamin Toxicity. Updated June 3, 2013. Medscape Web site. http://emedicine.medscape.com/article/819426-overview. Accessed August 15, 2014.
14. Centers for Disease Control and Prevention. You Wear It Well: Wear Red and Lower Your Risk for Heart Disease. CDC Web site: http://www.cdc.gov/women/heart/WearItWell.pdf. Accessed February 23, 2012.
15. Yusuf S, Hawken S, Ounpuu S, et al. INTERHEART Study Investigators. Effect of potentially modifiable risk factors associated with myocardial infarction in 52 countries (the INTERHEART study): case-control study. *The Lancet*. 2004;364(9438):937-952.

Chapter 2

1. Hyman M. Why Treating Your Symptoms is a Recipe for Disaster. Updated September 12, 2012. DrHyman Web site. http://drhyman.com/why-treating-your-symptoms-is-a-recipe-for-disaster-3520/. Accessed February 23, 2012.

2. Schiff GD, Galanter WL, Duhig J, et al. Principles of conservative prescribing. *Arch Intern Med.* 2011;171(16):1433-1440. Available at: http://archinte.jamanetwork.com/article.aspx?articleid=1105913. Accessed February 23, 2012.
3. Board of Naturopathic Medicine. Naturopathy. Oregon Board of Naturopathic Medicine Web site. http://www.oregon.gov/obnm/pages/aboutnaturopathy.aspx. Accessed February 26, 2012.
4. Schauss AG. Let the Science and Evidence Guide Decision-Making on Vitamin D for the Benefit of Patients. *Natural Medicine Journal.* 2010. http://www.naturalmedicinejournal.net/home schauss.shtml. Accessed February 26, 2012.
5. Albert PJ, Proal AD, Marshall TG. Vitamin D: the alternative hypothesis. *Autoimmun Rev.* 2009;8(8):639-644.
6. Galland L. Drug-Supplement Interactions: the Good, the Bad and the Uncertain. IFM Symposium: Spotlight on Gut-Brain-Skin Theory. August 2013 Institute for Functional Medicine. www.functionalmedicine.org. [members-only access]

Chapter 3

1. Weatherby C. Lighten Up to Lose Health Woes and Weight? Vital Choice newsletter. March 3, 2011. Available at: http://www.vitalchoice.com/shop/pc/articlesView.asp?id=1303. Accessed February 26, 2012.
2. Adams CE, Leary MR. Promoting Self-Compassionate Attitudes Toward Eating Among Restrictive and Guilty Eaters. *J Soc Clin Psychol.* 2007;26(10):1120–1144.
3. Neff KD, Rude SS, Kirkpatrick KL. An examination of self-compassion in relation to positive psychological functioning and personality traits. *J of Research in Personality.* 2007;41(4):908-916.
4. Hyman M. Food Addiction: Could it Explain Why 70 Percent of Americans are Fat? October 18, 2011. Dr. Hyman Web Site. http://drhyman.com/blog/conditions/food-addiction-could-it-explain-why-70-percent-of-america-is-fat/. Accessed February 14, 2011.
5. Snyder MA. *The Full Diet: A Weight-Loss Doctor's 7-day Guide to Shedding Pounds for Good.* Carlsbad, CA: Hay House Publishing; 2012.

6. Amen DG. *Change Your Brain, Change Your Life: The Breakthrough Program for Conquering Anxiety, Depression, Obsessiveness, Anger, and Impulsiveness.* New York, NY: Harmony Publishing; 1999.
7. Northrup C. Opening your heart to summer. Flourish Radio Show, Hayhouse Radio. July 6, 2011. http://www.hayhouseradio.com/#!/episode/opening-your-heart-to-summer-7456. Accessed February 23, 2012.
8. Ruuskanen A, Kaukinen K, Collin P, et al. Positive serum antigliadin antibodies without celiac disease in the elderly population: does it matter? *Scand J Gastroenterol.* 2010;45(10):1197-1202.
9. Vojdani A. Inflammation & Mood Disorders. The Mucosal Barrier Function Test [teleseminar]. September, 2009. Functional Medicine Seminars. Sponsored by BioHealth Laboratory.
10. Shor DB, Barzilai O, Ram M, et al. Gluten sensitivity in multiple sclerosis: experimental myth or clinical truth? *Ann N Y Acad Sci.* 2009;1173:343-349.
11. Mercola J. 3 Ounces of Wheat a Day May Be Harming Your Brain. July 4, 2011. Mercola Web site. http://articles.mercola.com/sites/articles/archive/2011/07/04/can-eating-this-common-grain-cause-psychiatric-problems.aspx. Accessed February 23, 2012.
12. Dickerson F, Stallings C, Origoni A, et al. Markers of gluten sensitivity and celiac disease in recent-onset psychosis and multi-episode schizophrenia. *Biol Psychiatry.* 2010;68(1):100-104.
13. Dohan FC, Harper EH, Clark MH, et al. Is schizophrenia rare if grain is rare? *Biol Psychiatry.* 1984;19(3):385-399.
14. Hyman M. Why Antidepressants Don't Work for Treating Depression. *Huffington Post.* April 24, 2010. Available at: http://www.huffingtonpost.com/dr-mark-hyman/depression-medication-why_b_550098.html. Accessed February 23, 2012.
15. Ilardi S. The Depression Cure: how to beat depression without drugs. *Psychology Today.* July 23, 2009. Available at: http://www.psychologytoday.com/blog/the-depression-cure. Accessed February 23, 2012.
16. Mercola J. Doctor Warns: Eat Soy and You'll Look 5 Years Older. Mercola Web site. December 8, 2011. http://articles.mercola.com/sites/articles/archive/2011/12/08/the-dirty-little-secret-hidden-in-much-of-your-health-food.aspx?e_cid=20111208_DNL_art_3. Accessed February 26, 2012.
17. Balk E, Chung M, Chew P, et al. The Effects of Soy on Health Outcomes. Agency for Healthcare Research and Quality (US). *AHRQ Evidence Reports/*

      Technology Assessments. Aug 2005;126. Available at: http://www.ncbi.nlm.nih.gov/books/NBK37881/. Accessed February 23, 2012.

[18] Mercola J. How to Starve Cancer Out of Your Body - Avoid These Top 4 Cancer-Feeding Foods. January 14, 2012. Mercola Web site. http://articles.mercola.com/sites/articles/archive/2012/01/14/dr-christine-horner-interview.aspx?e_cid=20120114_DNL_art_1. Accessed February 23, 2012.

[19] Enig M, Fallon S. Teens Before Their Time. September 8, 2002. The Weston A. Price Foundation Web site. http://www.westonaprice.org/soy-alert/teens-before-their-time. Accessed February 23, 2012.

[20] Gaby A. Controversies in Nutrition. Talk By Topic [presentation]. January, 2012. Institute for Functional Medicine Web site. www.functionalmedicine.org. [members-only access] Accessed February 26, 2012.

Chapter 4

[1] Lamm B. *Just 10 Lbs: Ten Easy Steps to Weighing What You Want (Finally!).* Carlsbad, CA: Hay House, Inc. January 2011.

[2] Rosenbaum M, Sy M, Povlovich K, et al. Leptin reverses weight loss–induced changes in regional neural activity responses to visual food stimuli. *J Clin Invest.* 2008;118(7):2583-2591.

[3] Stice E, Spoor S, Bohon C, et al. Relation of reward from food intake and anticipated food intake to obesity: a functional magnetic resonance imaging study. *J Abnorm Psychol.* 2008;117(4):924-935.

[4] Yang Q. Gain weight by "going diet?" Artificial sweeteners and the neurobiology of sugar cravings. Neuroscience 2010. *Yale J Biol Med.* 2010;83(2):101-108. Available at: http://www.ncbi.nlm.nih.gov/pmc/articles/PMC2892765/. Accessed February 26, 2012.

[5] Mercola J. Exercise Can Override "Fat Genes." September 16, 2010. Mercola Web site. http://fitness.mercola.com/sites/fitness/archive/2010/09/16/exercise-can-override-fat-genes.aspx. Accessed February 23, 2012. Original Source: Hellmich N. Exercise can override 'fat genes,' study finds. *USA Today.* August 31, 2011. http://usatoday30.usatoday.com/yourlife/fitness/exercise/2010-09-01-fatgenes01_ST_N.htm. Accessed February 26, 2012.

[6] Centers for Disease Control and Prevention. Obesity at a Glance: Halting the Epidemic by Making Health Easier. 2009. CDC Web site. http://www.

cdc.gov/nccdphp/publications/AAG/pdf/obesity.pdf. Accessed February 23, 2012.

7   Carroll M, Curtin L, Flegal K, Ogden C. Prevalence and trends in obesity among US adults, 1999-2008. *JAMA* 2010;303(3):235-241. Available at: https://carmenwiki.osu.edu/download/attachments/26513653/JAMA+2008+Obesity+Trends.pdf. Accessed February 23, 2012.

8   The National Heart, Lung, and Blood Institute. Rationale. NHLBI Web site. https://www.nhlbi.nih.gov/health-pro/guidelines/current/obesity-guidelines/e textbook/ratnl/20.htm. Accessed February 23, 2012.

9   D'Adamo PJ. Blood Group Genetics, Exercise and Stress. 2008-2010. Eat Right for Your Type®: Official Website of Dr. Peter D'Adamo and the Blood Type Diet. http://www.dadamo.com/science stress exercise.htm. Accessed October 23, 2013.

10 Quasarano A. Spotlight – Des Depass: Exercise Right 4 Your Type®. January 2011. Eat Right for Your Type®. D'Adamo Personalized Nutrition® Newsletter. 2010;7(12). Eat Right for Your Type® Web site. https://www.4yourtype.com/NEWSLETTER 8 1.asp#spotlight. Accessed October 23, 2013.

11 Science Daily. Yoga boosts stress-busting hormone, reduces pain, study finds. *ScienceDaily*. July 27, 2011. Available at: http://www.sciencedaily.com/releases/2011/07/110727131421.htm. Accessed February 23, 2012.

12 The Chopra Center Newsletter. Let Go of Stress and Struggle: Embrace the Law of Least Effort. Chopra Web site. August 2011. http://www.chopra.com/files/newsletter/Aug11/Newsletter-Aug11-yoga.html. Accessed February 23, 2012.

13 Korpela KM, Ylén M, Tyrväinen L, Silvennoinen H. Favorite green, waterside and urban environments, restorative experiences and perceived health in Finland. *Health Promot Int.* 2010;25(2):200-209.

14 Woodcock J, Franco OH, Orsini N, Roberts I. Non-vigorous physical activity and all-cause mortality: systematic review and meta-analysis of cohort studies. *Int J Epidemiol.* 2011;40(1):121-138.

Chapter 5

1   Hadjivassiliou M, Grünewald RA, Davies-Jones GB. Gluten sensitivity as a neurological illness. *J Neurol Neurosurg Psychiatry.* 2002;72(5):560-563

Available at: http://www.ncbi.nlm.nih.gov/pmc/articles/PMC1737870/pdf/v072p00560.pdf. Accessed February 23, 2012.

[2] Ji S. Opening Pandora's Bread Box: The Critical Role of Wheat Lectin in Human Disease. GreenMedInfo Web site. http://www.greenmedinfo.com/page/opening-pandoras-bread-box-critical-role-wheat-lectin-human-disease. Accessed February 23, 2012.

[3] American Academy of Allergy Asthma & Immunology. Food allergy: a practice parameter. 2006;96:S1-S68. AAAAI Web site. http://www.aaaai.org/Aaaai/media/MediaLibrary/PDF%20Documents/Practice%20and%20Parameters/food-allergy-2006.pdf. Accessed February 23, 2012.

[4] Shor DB, Barzilai O, Ram M, et al. Gluten sensitivity in multiple sclerosis: experimental myth or clinical truth? *Ann N Y Acad Sci.* 2009;1173:343-349.

[5] Farrell RJ, Kelly CP. Celiac Sprue. *N Engl J Med.* 2002;346(3):180-188. Available at: http://www.ucdenver.edu/academics/colleges/medicalschool/departments/medicine/Gastroenterology/Documents/Current%20Concepts%20-%20Celiac%20Sprue.pdf. Accessed February 26, 2012.

[6] Pynnönen PA, Isometsä ET, Verkasaloet MA, et al. Gluten-free diet may alleviate depressive and behavioural symptoms in adolescents with coeliac disease: a prospective follow-up case-series study. *BMC Psychiatry.* 2005;5:14.

[7] Kresser C. RHR: Pioneering Researcher Alessio Fasano, MD, on Gluten, Autoimmunity & Leaky Gut. Revolution Health Radio. 2012. ChrisKesser Web site. http://chriskresser.com/pioneering-researcher-alessio-fasano-m-d-on-gluten-autoimmunity-leaky-gut. Accessed May 24, 2014.

[8] Sapone A, Bai JC, Ciacci C, et al. Spectrum of gluten-related disorders: consensus on new nomenclature and classification. *BMC Med.* 2012;10:13.

[9] Ji S. The Dark Side of Wheat – New Perspectives on Celiac Disease and Wheat Intolerance. GreenMedInfo.com. Available at: http://www.greenmedinfo.com/page/dark-side-wheat-new-perspectives-celiac-disease-wheat-intolerance-sayer-ji. Accessed October 14, 2013.

[10] Ludvigsson JF, Montgomery SM, Ekbom A, et al. Small-intestinal histopathology and mortality risk in celiac disease. *JAMA.* 2009; 302(11):1171-1178.

[11] Chaitow L, Trenev L. Probiotics. Available at: http://www.holisticmed.com/detox/dtx-probio.txt. Accessed February 23, 2012.

12. Vael C, Verhulst SL, Nelen V, et al. Intestinal microflora and body mass index during the first three years of life: an observational study. *Gut Pathog.* 2011;3(1):8.
13. Diaz Heijtz R, Wang S, Anuar F, et al. Normal gut microbiota modulates brain development and behavior. *Proc Natl Acad Sci U S A.* 2011;108(7):3047-3052. Microbiome database at dr-lobisco.com

Chapter 6

1. National Institute of Mental Health. What is Depression? NIMH Web site. http://www.nimh.nih.gov/health/topics/depression/index.shtml. Accessed November 6, 2013.
2. Fournier JC, DeRubeis RJ, Hollon SD, et al. Antidepressant Drug Effects and Depression Severity: A Patient-Level Meta-analysis. *JAMA.* 2010;303(1):47-53.
3. Davis LJ. Five Reasons not to take SSRIs: Now that SSRIs don't work for depression, don't take them! Obsessively Yours. *Psychology Today.* January 7, 2010. Available at: http://www.psychologytoday.com/blog/obsessively-yours/201001/five-reasons-not-take-ssris. Accessed February 23, 2012.
4. Kirsch I, Deacon BJ, Huedo-Medina TB, et al. Initial severity and antidepressant benefits: a meta-analysis of data submitted to the Food and Drug Administration. *PLoS Med.* 2008;5(2):e45.
5. Paul M. Why Antidepressants Don't Work for So Many: Research finds cause of depression oversimplified, drugs aim at wrong target. October 23, 2009. Northwestern University Web site. http://www.northwestern.edu/newscenter/stories/2009/10/redei.html. Accessed November 7. 2013.
6. Fehér J, Kovács I, Balacco G, Gabrieli C. Role of gastrointestinal inflammations in the development and treatment of depression. *Orv Hetil.* 2011;152(37):1477-1485. [Article in Hungarian]
7. Nozaki C, Vergnano MA, Filliol D, et al. Zinc alleviates pain through high-affinity binding to the NMDA receptor NR2A subunit. *Nature Neurosci.* 2011;14(8):1017-1022.
8. Mischoulon D. The Science Behind Nutrients and Phytonutrients as Antidepressant Treatments. Talk By Topic [presentation]. February, 2012. Institute for Functional Medicine. www.functionalmedicine.org. [members-only access] Accessed February 26, 2012.

9. Amen D. *Change Your Brain, Change Your Life: The Breakthrough Program for Conquering Anxiety, Depression, Obsessiveness, Anger, and Impulsiveness.* New York, NY: Three Rivers Press; 1999.
10. Barth C, Villringer A, Sacher J. Sex hormones affect neurotransmitters and shape the adult female brain during hormonal transition periods. *Frontiers in Neuroscience.* 2015;9:37.
11. Uemura K, Shimada H, Doi T, Makizako H, et al. Depressive symptoms in older adults are associated with decreased cerebral oxygenation of the prefrontal cortex during a trail-making test. *Arch Gerontol Geriatr.* 2014 Sep-Oct;59(2):422-8.
12. Kumar V, Gill KD. Aluminum neurotoxicity: neurobehavioral and oxidative aspects. *Arch Toxicol.* 2009 Nov;83(11):965-78.
13. Fulgenzi A, Vietti D, Ferrero ME. Aluminum involvement in neurotoxicity. *Biomed Research International.* 2014; 2014: 758323 Available at: http://dx.doi.org/10.1155/2014/758323. Accessed December 14, 2015.
14. Abdollahi M1, Ranjbar A, Shadnia S, et al. Pesticides and oxidative stress: a review. *Med Sci Monit.* 2004 Jun;10(6):RA141-7.
15. Dayawansa S, Umeno K, Takakura H, et al. Autonomic responses during inhalation of natural fragrance of cedrol in humans. *Auton Neurosci.* 2003 Oct 31;108(1-2):79-86.
16. Kagawa D, Jokura H, Ochiai R, et al. The sedative effects and mechanism of action of cedrol inhalation with behavioral pharmacological evaluation. *Planta Med.* 2003 Jul;69(7):637-41.
17. Freidmann TS. Attention deficit and hyperactivity disorder (ADHD). Case Study. 1999-2001. Available at: http://files.meetup.com/1481956/ADHD%20Research%20by%20Dr.%20Terry%20Friedmann.pdf
18. Cho Mi-Y, Min ES, Hur, M-H, et al. Effects of Aromatherapy on the anxiety, vital signs, and sleep quality of percutaneous coronary intervention patients in intensive care units. *Evid Based Complement Alternat Med.* 2013; 2013: 381381.
19. Costa CA, Cury TC, Cassettari BO, et al. Citrus aurantium L. essential oil exhibits anxiolytic-like activity mediated by 5-HT(1A)-receptors and reduces cholesterol after repeated oral treatment. *BMC Complement Altern Med.* 2013 Feb 23;13:42.
20. Choi SY, Kang P, Lee HS, et al. Effects of inhalation of essential oil of *Citrus aurantium* L. var. *amara* on menopausal symptoms, stress, and estrogen

in postmenopausal women: a randomized controlled trial. *Evidence-based Complementary and Alternative Medicine.* 2014;2014:796518.

21. Kim S, Kim H-J, Yeo J-S, et al. The effect of lavender oil on stress, bispectral index values, and needle insertion pain in volunteers. *J Altern Complement Med.* 2011;17(9):823-826.

22. Oliff H. Lavender oil inhalation prior to surgery-like setting reduces perceptions of stress and pain. American Botanical Council. *HerbalGram.* 2011; 92(39).

23. Oriff H. Review of studies assessing the effect of lavender on anxiety. American Botanical Council. HerbalGram. August 8 2012; Herbal Clip Online:# 051254-454.

24. Oriff H Lavender-scented bath oil promotes sleep and reduces stress in infants. American Botanical Council. HerbalGram. July 8, 2008; Herbal Clip Online:# 020685-356.

25. Matsumoto T, Asakura H, Hayashi T. Does lavender aromatherapy alleviate premenstrual emotional symptoms?: a randomized crossover trial. *Biopsychosocial Medicine.* 2013;7:12.

26. Schreiner O. The Sesquiterpenes: a Monograph. [master's thesis]. Madison, WI. University of Wisconsin. Pharmaceutical Review Pub. Co. January 1, 1904.

27. Xu J, Guo Y, Zhao P, et al. Four new sesquiterpenes from *Commiphora myrrha* and their neuroprotective effects. *Fitoterapia.* 2012 Jun;83(4):801-5.

28. Xu J, Guo Y, Li Y, Zhao P, et al. Sesquiterpenoids from the resinous exudates of *Commiphora myrrha* and their neuroprotective effects. *Planta Med.* 2011 Dec;77(18):2023-8.

29. Neganova ME, Afanas'eva SV, Klochkov SG, et al. Mechanisms of antioxidant effect of natural sesquiterpene lactone and alkaloid derivatives. (abstract). *Bull Exp Biol Med.* 2012 Apr;152(6):720-2.

30. Wu XS, Xie T, Lin J, et al. An investigation of the ability of elemene to pass through the blood-brain barrier and its effect on brain carcinomas. (abstract) *J Pharm Pharmacol.* 2009 Dec;61(12):1653-6.

31. Inouye S. Abe S. Predominant adsorption of sesquiterpene constituents of lavender, tea tree, lemongrass and thyme thymol oils on hairless mouse and human hairs in an aromatic bath. *International Journal of Aromatherapy.* 2006; 16(2): 75-83.

32. Oluwatuyi M, Kaatz GW, Gibbons S. Antibacterial and resistance modifying activity of Rosmarinus officinalis. *Phytochemistry*. 2004 Dec;65(24):3249-54.
33. Korkina L, Kostyuk V, De Luca C, et al. Plant phenylpropanoids as emerging anti-inflammatory agents. *Mini Rev Med Chem*. 2011 Sep;11(10):823-835.
34. Nazzaro F, Fratianni F, De Martino L, et al. Effect of essential oils on pathogenic bacteria. *Pharmaceuticals*. 2013;6(12):1451-1474
35. Bayala B, Bassole IH, Scifo R, et al. Anticancer activity of essential oils and their chemical components – a review. *American Journal of Cancer Research*. 2014;4(6):591-607.
36. Linus Pauling Institute. Micronutrient Information Center. Cognitive Function. Oregon State University Web site. http://lpi.oregonstate.edu/mic/micronutrients-health/cognitive-function. Accessed December 17, 2015.
37. D'Silva S, Poscablo C, Habousha R, et al. Mind-body medicine therapies for a range of depression severity: a systematic review. *Psychosomatics*. 2012 Sep-Oct;53(5):407-23.
38. Church D, De Asis M, Brooks AJ. Brief group intervention using EFT (Emotional Freedom Techniques) for depression in college students: A randomized controlled trial. *Depression Research & Treatment*, 2012. doi:10.1155/2012/257172.
39. Muszyńska B, Łojewski M, Rojowski J, et al K. Natural products of relevance in the prevention and supportive treatment of depression. *Psychiatr Pol*. 2015 May-Jun;49(3):435-53. doi: 10.12740/PP/29367.
40. *Essential Oils Desk Reference*. 4th ed. USA: Essential Science Publishing; 2007.
41. Young G. *Essential Oils Integrative Medical Guide*. 2nd ed. Canandaigua, NY: Life Sciences Press; 2003.
42. Higley C, Higley A. *Reference Guide for Essential Oils*. Spanish Fork, UT: Abundant Health; 2007.
43. Djilani, A & Dicko, A. *The Therapeutic Benefits of Essential Oils, Nutrition, Well-Being and Health*. Dr. Jaouad Bouayed ed. 2012; 160.
44. Koulivand PH, Khaleghi Ghadiri M, Gorji A. Lavender and the nervous system. *Evidence-based Complementary and Alternative Medicine: eCAM*. 2013;2013:681304.
45. Ali B, Al-Wabel NA, Shams S, et al. Essential oils used in aromatherapy: a systemic review. *Asian Pacific Journal of Tropical Biomedicine*. August 2015; 5(8): 601-611.

46. Zabirunnisa M, Gadagi JS, Gadde P, et al. Dental patient anxiety: possible deal with *Lavender* fragrance. *Journal of Research in Pharmacy Practice*. 2014;3(3):100-103.
47. Alanko K. Aromatherapists. In: Kanerva L, Wahlberg JE, Elsner P, Maibach HI, eds. *Handbook of Occupational Dermatology*. Heidelberg, NY. Springer Berlin Heidelberg; 2000: 811-813.
48. Ju MS, Lee S, Bae I, Hur MH, et al. Effects of aroma massage on home blood pressure, ambulatory blood pressure, and sleep quality in middle-aged women with hypertension. *Evid Based Complement Alternat Med*. 2013;2013:403251.
49. Pemberton E, Turpin PG. The effect of essential oils on work-related stress in intensive care unit nurses. *Holist Nurs Pract*. 2008;22(2):97-102. Available at: http://www.kgstiles.com/ResearchStudyStressICUNursesUsingLavender%26ClarySageEssentialOilsPubDateSpring2008.pdf. Accessed October 15, 2013.
50. University of Maryland Medical Center (UMMC). Complementary and Alternative Medicine Guide. Herb. Valerian. UNMC Web site: http://umm.edu/health/medical/altmed/herb/valerian. Accessed December 29, 2015.
51. Yurcheshen M, Seehuus M, Pigeon W. Updates on nutraceutical sleep therapeutics and investigational research. *Evidence-based Complementary and Alternative Medicine : eCAM*. 2015;2015:105256.
52. Anderson G, Elmer GW, Taibi DM, et al. Pharmacokinetics of valerenic acid after single and multiple doses of valerian in Older women. *Phytotherapy Research*. 2010: 24:1442–1446.
53. Fernández-San-Martín MI, Masa-Font R, Palacios-Soler L, et al. Effectiveness of Valerian on insomnia: a meta-analysis of randomized placebo-controlled trials. *Sleep Medicine*. 2010;11(6):505–511.
54. Dietz BM, Mahady GB, Pauli G., et al. Valerian extract and valerenic acid are partial agonists of the $5-HT_{5a}$ receptor in vitro. *Molecular Brain Research*. 2005;138(2):191–197.
55. Müller CE, Schumacher B, Brattström A., Abourashed EA, et al. Interactions of valerian extracts and a
56. Hadley S, Petry JJ. Valerian. *Am Fam Physician*. 2003 Apr 15;67(8):1755-1758.
57. Gromball J, Beschorner F, Wantzen C, Paulsen U, et al. Hyperactivity, concentration difficulties and impulsiveness improve during seven weeks'

treatment with valerian root and lemon balm extracts in primary school children. *Phytomedicine*. July-August 2014. 21(8-9): 1098-1103.

58   Costa CA, Cury TC, Cassettari BO, Takahira RK, et al. *Citrus aurantium* L. essential oil exhibits anxiolytic-like activity mediated by 5-HT(1A)-receptors and reduces cholesterol after repeated oral treatment. *BMC Complement Altern Med*. 2013 Feb 23;13:42.

59   Azanchi T, Shafaroodi H, Asgarpanah J. Anticonvulsant activity of *Citrus aurantium* blossom essential oil (neroli): involvement of the GABAergic system. *Nat Prod Commun*. 2014 Nov;9(11):1615-8.

60   Namazi M, Amir Ali Akbari S, Mojab F, et al Aromatherapy with Citrus aurantium oil and anxiety during the first stage of labor. *Iranian Red Crescent Medical Journal*. 2014;16(6):e18371.

61   Ammar AH, Bouajila J, Lebrihi A, et al. Chemical composition and in vitro antimicrobial and antioxidant activities of *Citrus aurantium* l. flowers essential oil (Neroli oil). *Pak J Biol Sci*. 2012 Nov 1;15(21):1034-40.

62   Sarrou E, Chatzopoulou P, Dimassi-Theriou K, et al. Volatile constituents and antioxidant activity of peel, flowers and leaf oils of *Citrus aurantium* L. growing in Greece. *Molecules*. 2013 Sep 2;18(9):10639-47.

63   d'Alessio PA, Ostan R, Bisson JF, et al. Oral administration of d-limonene controls inflammation in rat colitis and displays anti-inflammatory properties as diet supplementation in humans. *Life Sci*. 2013;92(24-26):1151–6.

Chapter 7

1   Nussey S, Whitehead S. Endocrinology: An Integrated Approach. Oxford: BIOS Scientific Publishers; 2001. Chapter 1, Principles of endocrinology. Available from: http://www.ncbi.nlm.nih.gov/books/NBK20/

2   University of Michigan. Characteristics of Chemical Messengers. Chapter 1. Available at: https://www.google.com/url?sa=t&rct=j&q=&esrc=s&source=web&cd=6&ved=0ahUKEwiBwM7-uevJAhUGVyYKHcNTA6AQFgg8MAU&url=http%3A%2F%2Fwww.umich.edu%2F~kcourses%2Fw99%2Fmvs442%2Fchapter1.pdf&usg=AFQjCNGh1LSaNNP8TKYWjAz2Odl77kEzpg&cad=rja

3   De Vito P. Atrial natriuretic peptide: an old hormone or a new cytokine? *Peptides*. 2014 Aug;58:108-16.

4. Lovejoy JC. The influence of sex hormones on obesity across the female life span (abstract). *J Women's Health*. 1998 Dec;7(10):1247-56.
5. Santini F, Marzullo P, Rotondi M, et al. Mechanisms in endocrinology: the crosstalk between thyroid gland and adipose tissue: signal integration in health and disease. *Eur J Endocrinol*. October 1, 2014.
6. MA, Hogan PE, Fineberg SE, Howard G, Schrott H, Waclawiw MA, Bush TL. Effect of postmenopausal hormone therapy on glucose and insulin concentrations. PEPI investigators. Postmenopausal estrogen/progestin interventions. *Diabetes Care*. 1998 Oct;21(10):1589-95.
7. Karar T, Alhammad RIS, Fattah MA, Alanazi A, Qureshi S. Relation between glycosylated hemoglobin and lipid and thyroid hormone among patients with type 2 diabetes mellitus at King Abdulaziz Medical City, Riyadh. *Journal of Natural Science, Biology, and Medicine*. 2015;6(1): S75-S79.
8. Bhatia A, Sekhorn HK, Bhatia GK. Sex hormones and immune dimorphism. *The Scientific World Journal*. 2014; 159150.
9. Hampl R, Bičíková M, Sosvorová L. How hormones influence composition and physiological function of the brain-blood barrier. *Physiol Res*. 2015;64(2):S259-64.
10. Shepherd JE. Effects of estrogen on cognition, mood, and degenerative brain diseases. *J Am Pharm Assoc (Wash)*. 2001 Mar-Apr;41(2):221-8.
11. Hautanen A. Synthesis and regulation of sex hormone-binding globulin in obesity. *Int J Obes Relat Metab Disord*. 2000 Jun;24(2):S64-70.
12. Knochenhauer ES, Boots LR, Potter HD, Azziz R. Differential binding of estradiol and testosterone to SHBG. Relation to circulating estradiol levels. *J Reprod Med*. 1998 Aug;43(8):665-70.
13. Santin AP, Furlanetto TW. Role of estrogen in thyroid function and growth regulation. *Journal of Thyroid Research*. 2011;2011:875125.
14. Holtorf K. Thyroid hormone transport into cellular tissue. *Journal of Restorative Medicine*. April 2014; 3(1): 53-68.
15. Brito JP, Gionfriddo MR, Nofal A, et al. The accuracy of thyroid nodule ultrasound to predict thyroid cancer: systematic review and meta-analysis. *The Journal of Clinical Endocrinology and Metabolism*. 2014;99(4):1253-1263.
16. Ranabir S, Reetu K. Stress and hormones. *Indian Journal of Endocrinology and Metabolism*. 2011;15(1):18-22.
17. Simpson ER. Sources of estrogen and their importance. *J Steroid Biochem Mol Biol*. 2003 Sep;86(3-5):225-30.

18. Jerjes WK, Taylor N, Peters T, Wessely S, Cleare AJ. Urinary cortisol and cortisol metabolite excretion in chronic fatigue syndrome. *Psychosomatic Medicine*. 2006 Jul; 68(4):578-82.
19. Klachko DM, Johnson ER. The liver and circulating thyroid hormones. *J Clin Gastroenterol*. 1983 Oct;5(5):465-71.
20. Yang HP, Gonzalez Bosquet J, Li Q, Platz E, et al. Common genetic variation in the sex hormone metabolic pathway and endometrial cancer risk: pathway-based evaluation of candidate genes. *Carcinogenesis*. 2010;31(5):827-833.
21. Levy S. Estrogen metabolite ratio testing: is it worthwhile? American Board of Integrative Holistic Medicine. March 10, 2013. Available at: http://www.abihm.org/estrogen-metabolite-ratio-testing-is-it-worthwhile
22. Fuhrman BJ, Schairer C, Gail MH, et al. Estrogen metabolism and risk of breast cancer in postmenopausal women. *J Natl Cancer Ist*. 2012 Feb 22;104(4):326-39.
23. Schor J. Estrogen metabolite ratios: time for us to let go. *Townsend Letter*. January 2013. Available at: http://www.townsendletter.com/Jan2013/estrogen0113.html. Accessed May 2015.
24. Dunning AM, Dowsett M, Healey CS, et al. Polymorphisms associated with circulating sex hormone levels in postmenopausal women. *JNCI J Natl Cancer Inst*. 2004; 96 (12): 936-945.
25. Sørensen HG, van der Deure WM, Hansen PS, et al. Identification and consequences of polymorphisms in the thyroid hormone receptor alpha and beta genes. *Thyroid*. 2008 Oct;18(10):1087-94.
26. Doll H, Brown S, Thurston A, Vessey M. Pyridoxine (vitamin B6) and the premenstrual syndrome: a randomized crossover trial. *The Journal of the Royal College of General Practitioners*. 1989;39(326):364-368.
27. American Thyroid Association. General Information/Press Room. ATA Web site. http://www.thyroid.org/media-main/about-hypothyroidism/. Accessed December 20, 2015.
28. The National Institute of Diabetes and Digestive and Kidney Diseases. Hypothyroidism. NIDDK Web site. http://www.niddk.nih.gov/health-information/health-topics/endocrine/hypothyroidism/Pages/fact-sheet.aspx. Accessed December 20, 2015.
29. Nussey S, Whitehead S. *Endocrinology: An Integrated Approach*. Oxford: BIOS Scientific Publishers; 2001. Chapter 3, The thyroid gland. Available from: http://www.ncbi.nlm.nih.gov/books/NBK28/

30. Ranabir S, Reetu K. Stress and hormones. *Indian Journal of Endocrinology and Metabolism*. 2011;15(1):18-22. doi:10.4103/2230-8210.77573.
31. American Psychological Association. Stress Effects on the Body. APA Web site. http://www.apa.org/helpcenter/stress-body.aspx. Accessed December 20, 2015.
32. Whirledge S, Cidlowski JA. Glucocorticoids, Stress, and Fertility. *Minerva endocrinologica*. 2010;35(2):109-125.
33. Chao A, Grilo CM, White MA, Sinha R. Food cravings mediate the relationship between chronic stress and body mass index. *J Health Psychol*. 2015 Jun;20(6):721-9.
34. Seck-Gassama, Ndoye O, Mbodj M, Akala, et al. Serum cortisol level variations in thyroid diseases. [Article in French]. *Dakar Med*. 2000;45(1):30-3.
35. Hussain D. Stress, immunity, and health: research findings and implications. *International Journal of Psychosocial Rehabilitation*. 2010;15(1) 94-100.
36. Segerstrom SC, Miller GE. Psychological stress and the human immune system: a meta-analytic study of 30 years of inquiry. *Psychological bulletin*. 2004;130(4):601-630.
37. Innes KE, Vincent HK, Taylor AG, et al. Chronic stress and insulin resistance–related indices of cardiovascular disease. Part I. *Altern Ther Health Med*. 2007;13(4):46-52.
38. Abercrombie HC, Jahn AL, Davidson RJ, et al. Cortisol's effects on hippocampal activation in depressed patients are related to alterations in memory formation. *Journal of psychiatric research*. 2011;45(1):15-23.
39. Vythilingam M, Vermetten E, Anderson GM, et al. Hippocampal volume, memory, and cortisol status in major depressive disorder: effects of treatment. *Biol Psychiatry*. 2004 Jul 15;56(2):101-12.
40. Lupien SJ, de Leon M, de Santi S, et al. Cortisol levels during human aging predict hippocampal atrophy and memory deficits. *Nat Neurosci*. 1998 May;1(1):69-73.
41. Lindauer RJ, Olff M, van Meijel EP, et al. Cortisol, learning, memory, and attention in relation to smaller hippocampal volume in police officers with posttraumatic stress disorder. *Biol Psychiatry*. 2006 Jan 15;59(2):171-7.
42. Center for Disease Control and Prevention. Ace Study: Major Findings. CDC Web Site: http://www.cdc.gov/violenceprevention/acestudy/findings.html. Accessed December 22, 2015

43. Nash G. Q & A: Depression, Stress, and Your Blood Type. D'Adamo Personalized Nutrition® Newsletter. 2010;7(12). Eat Right for Your Type® Web site. https://www.4yourtype.com/NEWSLETTER_7_12.asp. Accessed February 26, 2012.
44. Gore VA, Chappell SE, Benton JA, et al. Executive Summary to EDC-2: The Endocrine Society's Second Scientific Statement on Endocrine-Disrupting Chemicals. *Endocrine Reviews.* 2015; er.2015-1093.
45. Diamanti-Kandarakis E, Bourguignon J-P, Giudice LC, et al. Endocrine-disrupting chemicals: an Endocrine Society Scientific Statement. *Endocr Rev.* 2009; 30(4): 293–342.
46. Bjørnerem A, Straume B, Midtby M, et al. Endogenous sex hormones in relation to age, sex, lifestyle factors, and chronic diseases in a general population: the Tromsø Study. *J Clin Endocrinol Metab.* 2004 Dec;89(12):6039-47.
47. Allen NE, Appleby PN, Davey GK, et al. Lifestyle and nutritional determinants of bioavailable androgens and related hormones in British men. *Cancer Causes Control.* 2002 May;13(4):353-63.
48. Baker FC, Driver HS. Circadian rhythms, sleep, and the menstrual cycle. *Sleep Med.* 2007 Sep;8(6):613-22.
49. Konieczna A, Rutkowska A1, Rachoń D. Health risk of exposure to Bisphenol A (BPA). *Rocz Panstw Zakl Hig.* 2015;66(1):5-11.
50. Brown SG, Morrison LA, Calibuso MJ, Christiansen TM. The menstrual cycle and sexual behavior: relationship to eating, exercise, sleep and health patterns. *Women & health.* 2008;48(4):429-444.
51. Iurescia S, Seripa D, Rinaldi M. Role of the 5-HTTLPR and SNP promoter polymorphisms on serotonin transporter gene expression: a closer look at genetic architecture and in vitro functional studies of common and uncommon allelic variants. *Mol Neurobiol.* 2015 Oct 13.
52. Boulour S, Braunstein G. Testosterone therapy in women: a review. *International Journal of Impotence Research.* 2005 May; 17, 399–408.
53. Reynisdottir S, Langin D, Carlström K, et al. Effects of weight reduction on the regulation of lipolysis in adipocytes of women with upper-body obesity. *Clin Sci (Lond).* 1995 Oct;89(4):421-9.
54. Corbould A. Effects of androgens on insulin action in women: is androgen excess a component of female metabolic syndrome? *Diabetes Metab Res Rev.* 2008 Oct;24(7):520-32.

55. Ziv-Gal A, Flaws JA. Factors that may influence the experience of hot flushes by healthy middle-aged women. *Journal of Women's Health.* 2010;19(10):1905-1914.
56. Kronenberg F, Cote LJ, Linkie DM, et al. Menopausal hot flashes: thermoregulatory, cardiovascular, and circulating catecholamine and LH changes. *Maturitas.* 1984 Jul;6(1):31-43.
57. Reichrath J, Lehmann B, Carlberg C, et al. Vitamins as hormones. *Horm Metab Res.* 2007 Feb;39(2):71-84.
58. Chen C-L, Tetri LH, Neuschwander-Tetri BA, et al. A Mechanism by Which Dietary Trans Fats Cause Atherosclerosis. *The Journal of nutritional biochemistry.* 2011;22(7):649-655.
59. Lopez-Garcia E1, Schulze MB, Meigs JB, et al. Consumption of trans fatty acids is related to plasma biomarkers of inflammation and endothelial dysfunction. *J Nutr.* 2005 Mar;135(3):562-6.
60. Vanevski F, Xu B. Molecular and neural bases underlying roles of BDNF in the control of body weight. *Frontiers in Neuroscience.* 2013;7:37.
61. Anderton MJ, Manson MM, Verschoyle R, et al. Physiological Modeling of Formulated and Crystalline 3,3'-Diindolythmethane pharmacokinetics following oral administration in mice. *Drug Met & Disposition.* June 2004; 32 (6) 632-638.
62. Reed GA, Arneson DW, Putnam WC, et al. Single-Dose and Multiple-Dose Administration of Indole-3-Carbinol to Women: Pharmacokinetics Based on 3,3'-Diindolylmethane. *Cancer Epidemiol Biomarkers Prev.* December 2006 15; 2477.
63. Patisaul HB, Jefferson W. The pros and cons of phytoestrogens. *Frontiers in neuroendocrinology* 2010;31(4):400-419.
64. Chandrasekhar K, Kapoor J, Anishetty S. A prospective, randomized double-blind, placebo-controlled study of safety and efficacy of a high-concentration full-spectrum extract of *ashwagandha* root in reducing stress and anxiety in adults. *Indian Journal of Psychological Medicine.* 2012;34(3):255-262.
65. Conaway E. Bioidentical hormones: an evidence-based review for primary care providers. *J Am Osteopath Assoc.* 2011 Mar;111(3):153-64.
66. Innes KE, Selfe KT, Vishnu A. Mind-body therapies for menopausal symptoms: a systematic review. *Maturitas* 2010; 66(2): 135-149

67. Northrup C. *Women's Body Women's Wisdom*. New York, NY: Random House; 2010.

Chapter 8

1. Department of Health and Human Services. About NTP. 2015. National Toxicology Program Web site. http://ntp.niehs.nih.gov/about/index.html. Accessed December 23, 2015.
2. Department of Health and Human Services. Fourth National Report on Human Exposure to Environmental Chemicals. 2009. Centers for Disease Control and Prevention. http://www.cdc.gov/exposurereport/pdf/FourthReport.pdf. Accessed March 2010.
3. Marshall WJ, Bangert SK. Chapter 13: The assessment of hepatic function and investigation of jaundice. In: Marshall WJ, Bangert SK, ed. Clinical Biochemistry: Metabolic and Clinical Aspects. 2nd ed. Philadelphia, PA: Elsevier. 2008. 253-272.
4. Trasande L, Zoeller RT, Hass U, et al. Estimating burden and disease costs of exposure to endocrine-disrupting chemicals in the European Union. *The Journal of Clinical Endocrinology and Metabolism*. 2015;100(4):1245-1255.
5. Gore VA, Chappell SE, Benton JA, et al. Executive Summary to EDC-2: The Endocrine Society's Second Scientific Statement on Endocrine-Disrupting Chemicals. *Endocrine Reviews*. 2015; er.2015-1093.
6. Diamanti-Kandarakis, E, Bourguignon, J-P, Giudice, LC, et al. Endocrine-disrupting chemicals: an Endocrine Society Scientific Statement. *Endocr Rev*. 2009; 30(4): 293–342.
7. Stel J, Legler J. Early life exposure to obesogenic endocrine disrupting chemicals. *Endocrinology*. August 4, 2015. Available at: http://dx.doi.org/10.1210/en.2015-1434#sthash.vTafZbko.dpuf. Accessed November 23, 2015.
8. Mu D, Gao F, Fan Z, et al. Levels of phthalate metabolites in urine of pregnant women and risk of clinical pregnancy loss. *Sci. Technol.* 2015;49(17):10651–10657.
9. Ünüvar T, Büyükgebiz A. Fetal and neonatal endocrine disruptors. *Journal of Clinical Research in Pediatric Endocrinology*. 2012;4(2):51-60.
10. Houston M. The role of nutrition and nutraceutical supplements in the treatment of hypertension. *World Journal of Cardiology*. 2014;6(2):38-66.
11. Wright RO, Christiani D. Gene-environment interaction and children's health and development. *Current opinion in pediatrics*. 2010;22(2):197-201.

12. Pinto N, Dolan ME. Clinically Relevant Genetic Variations in Drug Metabolizing Enzymes. *Current drug metabolism*. 2011;12(5):487-497.
13. Zablotska LB, Chen Y, Graziano JH, et al. Protective effects of B vitamins and antioxidants on the risk of arsenic-related skin lesions in Bangladesh. *Environmental Health Perspectives*. 2008;116(8):1056-1062.
14. Cummins R. Put the Fat Cats on a Diet: Stop Buying Tainted Food From Billion Dollar Corporations. December 7, 2011. Organic Consumers Association Web site. http://www.organicconsumers.org/articles/article_24448.cfm. Accessed February 23, 2012.
15. Shapiro TA, Fahey JW, Wade KL, et al. Chemoprotective glucosinolates and isothiocyanates of broccoli sprouts: metabolism and excretion in humans. *Cancer Epidemiol Biomarkers Prev*. 2001;10(5):501-508. Available at: http://cebp.aacrjournals.org/content/10/5/501.long. Accessed February 23, 2012.
16. Liska D. The Detoxification Enzyme Systems. *Altern Med Rev*. 1998;3(3):187-198.
17. Weatherby C. Cocoa and Dark Chocolate May Aid Gut Health. Vital Choice newsletter. December 31, 2010. Available at: http://www.vitalchoice.com/shop/pc/articlesView.asp?id=1201. Accessed February 26, 2012.
18. Buitrago-Lopez A, Sanderson J, Johnson L, et al. Chocolate consumption is associated with a substantial reduction in the risk of cardiometabolic disorders. *BMJ*. 2011;343:d4488. Available at: http://www.bmj.com/content/343/bmj.d4488. Accessed February 23, 2012.
19. Environmental Working Group. Top Tips for Safer Products. EWGs Skin Deep Cosmetic Database. 2007-2015. EWG Web site: http://www.ewg.org/skindeep/top-tips-for-safer-products/#women. Accessed March 17, 2013.
20. Shehzad A, Ha T, Subhan F, Lee YS. New mechanisms and the anti-inflammatory role of curcumin in obesity and obesity-related metabolic diseases. *Eur J Nutr*. 2011;50(3):151-161.
21. Magistrelli A, Chezem JC. Effect of ground cinnamon on postprandial blood glucose concentration in normal-weight and obese adults. *J Acad Nutr Diet*. 2012;112(11):1806-9.
22. Khan A, Safdar M, Ali Khan MM, Khattak KN, Anderson RA. Cinnamon improves glucose and lipids of people with type 2 diabetes (abstract). *Diabetes Care*. 2003 Dec;26(12):3215-8.
23. Roussel AM1, Hininger I, Benaraba R, Ziegenfuss TN, Anderson RA. Antioxidant effects of a cinnamon extract in people with impaired

fasting glucose that are overweight or obese (abstract). *J Am Coll Nutr.* 2009;28(1):16-21

[24] Bursill CA, Roach PD. Modulation of cholesterol metabolism by the green tea polyphenol (-)-epigallocatechin gallate in cultured human liver (HepG2) cells (abstract). *J Agric Food Chem.* 2006 Mar 8;54(5):1621-6.

[25] Lee VS, Dou J, Chen RJ, et al. Oolong tea accumulates the flavonols myricetin, quercetin, and kaempferol, and high levels of gallic acid. *J Agric Food Chem.* 2008;56(17):7950-7956.

[26] Siddiqui MZ. Boswellia serrata, a potential antiinflammatory agent: an overview. *Indian J Pharm Sci.* 2011;73(3):255-261.

[27] Xia Z, Mao X, Luo Y. Study on antifungal mechanism of alpha-pinene. *Hunan Yi Ke Da Xue Xue Bao.* 1999;24(6):507-509. [Article in Chinese]

[28] DeNoon DJ. Expert Panel: Cell Phones Might Cause Brain Cancer. WebMD Web site. http://www.webmd.com/cancer/news/20110531/expert-panel-cell-phones-might-cause-brain-cancer. Accessed February 23, 2012.

[29] Karatsoreos IN, Bhagat S, Bloss EB, et al. Disruption of circadian clocks has ramifications for metabolism, brain, and behavior. *Proc Natl Acad Sci U S A.* 2011;108(4):1657-1662. PNAS Web site. http://www.pnas.org/content/108/4/1657.full. Accessed February 20, 2013.

[30] Cuypers K, Krokstaad S, Holmen TL, et al. Patterns of receptive and creative cultural activities and their association with perceived health, anxiety, depression and satisfaction with life among adults: the HUNT study, Norway. *J Epidemiol Community Health.* 2012;66(8):698-703.

[31] Martin FP, Rezzi S, Peré-Trepat E, et al. Metabolic effects of dark chocolate consumption on energy, gut microbiota, and stress-related metabolism in free-living subjects. *J Proteome Res.* 2009;8(12):5568-5579. Available at: http://www.ts-si.org/files/doi101021pr900607vpr900607v.pdf. Accessed June 13, 2014.

Chapter 9

[1] Cleveland Clinic. Heart Facts. Cleveland Clinic Web site. http://my.clevelandclinic.org/heart/heart-blood-vessels/heart-facts.aspx. Accessed August 28, 2013.

[2] February is American Heart Month. Healthy You Web site. http://www.healthyyouhmi.org/HEALTHY YOU Feature Stories/Feb feature.asp. Accessed February 23, 2012.

[3] Taylor F, Ward K, Moore TH, et al. Statins for the primary prevention of cardiovascular disease. *The Cochrane database of systematic reviews* 2011;(1):CD004816.

[4] Bankhead, C. Should Healthy People Take Statins? New Studies Say No. *Medpage Today*. June 28, 2010. Available at: http://www.medpagetoday.com/Cardiology/Prevention/20948. Accessed January 1, 2014.

[5] Petersen LK, Christensen K, Kragstrup J. Lipid-lowering treatment to the end? A review of observational studies and RCTs on cholesterol and mortality in 80+-year olds. *Age and Ageing*. 2010;39(6):674-680.

[6] Newman, D. Statins Given for 5 Years for Heart Disease Prevention (With Known Heart Disease). The NNT Group. November 2, 2013. Available at: http://www.thennt.com/nnt/statins-for-heart-disease-prevention-with-known-heart-disease/. Accessed January 1, 2015.

[7] Thavendiranathan P, Bagai A, Brookhart MA, Choudhry NK. Primary prevention of cardiovascular disease with statin therapy. *Arch Int Med*. 2006; 166: 2307-13.

[8] Baigent C, Keech A, Kearney PM, et al. Efficacy and safety of cholesterol-lowering treatment: prospective meta-analysis of data from 90,056 participants in 14 randomised trials of statins. Lancet. 2005;366(9493):1267-1278.

[9] Gutierrez J, Ramirez G, Rundek T, Sacco RL. Statin therapy in the prevention of recurrent cardiovascular events: a sex-based meta-analysis. *Arch Intern Med*. 2012 Jun 25;172(12):909-19.

[10] Hyman M. Why Women Should Stop Their Cholesterol-Lowering Medication. *Huffington Post*. January 20, 2012. Available at: http://www.huffingtonpost.com/dr-mark-hyman/women-cholesterol-medication b 1219496.html. Accessed February 23, 2012.

[11] Heffner KL, Waring ME, Roberts MB, et al. Social isolation, C-reactive protein, and coronary heart disease mortality among community-dwelling adults. *Soc Sci Med*. 2011;72(9):1482-1488.

[12] Mostofsky E, Maclure M, Sherword JB, et al. Risk of acute myocardial infarction after death of a significant person in one's life: the Determinants of Myocardial Infarction Onset Study. *Circulation*. 2012;125(3);491-496.

http://circ.ahajournals.org/content/125/3/491.long. Accessed February 23, 2012.

13. Mercola J. How Grief Can Break Your Heart. February 3, 2012. Mercola Web site. http://articles.mercola.com/sites/articles/archive/2012/02/03/how-grief-can-break-your-heart.aspx. Accessed February 23, 2012.

14. American Heart Association. Yoga and Heart Health. Updated April 10, 2014. AHA Web site. http://www.heart.org/HEARTORG/GettingHealthy/PhysicalActivity/Yoga-and-Heart-Health UCM 434966 Article.jsp#.TofOxRzXJs4. Accessed February 23, 2012.

INDEX

A

Adrenal gland support 101
antidepressant drugs 89
anxiety 39, 43, 63, 76, 82, 99, 100, 106, 107, 110, 119

B

blood sugar 35, 55

C

cardiovascular system 122
celiac disease 39, 42, 78, 80, 172
cholesterol 152
cleansing 135
conventional medicine 2, 6, 15, 17, 28, 128, 152
cortisol 63, 101, 115, 119, 120, 122, 126, 163, 164
cravings 33

D

depression 39, 43, 45, 63, 76, 87, 88, 89, 92, 93, 96, 100, 119, 176
detoxifying 135
diets 52

E

EMFs 143
epigenetics 164
essential oils
    mood 95
estrogen 47, 114, 119, 121, 123, 124, 126, 127, 128
evidence based medicine 11
exercise 57

F

functional medicine xiii, 24, 26, 27, 59, 62, 65, 68, 147

G

gastrointestinal xiii, 28, 38, 46, 47, 63, 68, 69, 72, 74, 75, 80, 82, 83, 93, 140, 165, 166, 176
gluten 38, 42, 44, 76, 77, 164, 172, 174, 175
gut-brain 34, 42, 70, 85

H

healthcare 2
holistic xv, 1, 13, 16, 28, 112
hormones 113, 114, 119

I

integrative medicine xvi, 2, 20, 24, 87

L

leaky gut 69

M

mal-absorption and intestinal permeability 69
mind-body medicine 27, 95, 129, 157

N

naturopathic medicine 6, 68
neurotransmitters 26, 36, 65, 68, 76, 85, 90, 91, 94, 95, 99, 118, 120, 126, 163, 165
nutrigenomics 6, 30, 62, 73
nutrition 36

O

organic 139

P

probiotics 80
progesterone 114, 115, 119, 121, 123, 126, 127, 128

S

safe cleansing supplements 140

T

thyroid 39, 41, 47, 94, 99, 101, 103, 115, 118, 119, 121, 124

W

weight loss 36, 52, 53, 54, 55, 58, 63, 64, 83, 134, 135, 138, 173

Made in the USA
Middletown, DE
02 March 2016